The
Anarchist AIDS
Medical Formulary

The
Anarchist AIDS
Medical Formulary

A Guide to
Guerrilla Immunology

Selected Essays
by
Charles R. Caulfield
with Billi Goldberg

North Atlantic Books
Berkeley, California

Notice to the Reader

This book is not intended to replace good medical diagnosis and treatment. Its purpose is to help you work with your health care practitioner in making informed treatment decisions.

The Anarchist AIDS Medical Formulary: A Guide to Guerrilla Immunology

Published by
North Atlantic Books
P.O. Box 12327
Berkeley, California 94701–9998

Cover and book design by Paula Morrison
Typeset by Catherine Campaigne
Printed in the United States of America by Malloy Lithography.

The Anarchist AIDS Medical Formulary is sponsored by The Society for the Study of Native Arts and Sciences, a nonprofit educational corporation whose goals are to develop an educational and crosscultural perspective linking various scientific, social, and artistic fields; to nurture a holistic view of arts, sciences, humanities, and healing; and to publish and distribute literature on the relationship of mind, body, and nature.

Library of Congress Cataloging-in-Publication Data
Caulfield, Charles R., 1956–
    The anarchist AIDS medical formulary : a guide to guerilla
immunology / Charles R. Caulfield with Billi Goldberg.
       p. cm.
    Includes bibliographical references.
    ISBN: 1-55643-175-9
    1. AIDS (Disease)—Alternative treatment.   I. Goldberg, Billi.
1934– . II. Title.
RC607.A263C383 1994
616. 97'92061—dc20   93-43598
                                      CIP

2   3   4   5   6   7   8   9 / 97 96 95 94

Acknowledgments

This collection of essays is dedicated to the memory
of Tom O'Connor, my friend, mentor,
and inspiration to keep fighting.
I consider it to be the logical continuation of his work.

Special thanks are due to the members of the Alternative Treatment Committee of ACT-UP San Francisco, H. Reg McDaniel, M.D., Raphael Stricker, M.D., Ray Chalker, Jim Henry, Blaine Elswood, John Page, D.D.S., Samuel Murdock, esq., Carol Mills, Sam Mather, and the late Terry Pulse, M.D., for providing support, encouragement, and light along the path.

Contents

Part Two: Alternative AIDS Treatments: Theories, Therapies, and Resources

Foreword

Have you known someone who died of AIDS? A relative, a friend, a neighbor? Most of us have. Do you know someone infected with the HIV virus? Most of us do. We think, of course, that they will die, that AIDS will kill them. We believe that their physical suffering may be alleviated somewhat by a variety of expensive drugs, whose alphabetic names—like AZT and ddI—have become commonplace.

The prevailing conventional wisdom tells us, and the best scientific minds in the world agree, that AIDS = Death, that AIDS entails a slow, agonizing progression of symptoms leading inevitably to the grave. That's the way it is.

Or is it?

Is restoration of a compromised immune system, even partial restoration, possible? And could it be affordable to all?

Ask these questions of most leading HIV researchers and medical practitioners, and they smile indulgently and say that they've heard it before. The miracle cures, the underground drugs, the treatment activists. They know all about it. Take your AZT and/or ddI, cash in your life insurance to pay for it, and wait to die. That's the way it is.

But is it?

By conventional reasoning, Charles Caulfield should be dead. Long dead. Buried a decade ago. Another of the seemingly endless AIDS statistics. In 1984, he was hospitalized with a then-rare form of pneumonia. There was no known treatment for what he had: the new disease that would eventually be named AIDS. It killed everybody who caught it.

But it didn't kill Caulfield. He survived. Back then, ten years ago, he was a nobody, just another guy carrying the weight of illness borne by all those who suffer from the so-called "gay disease." What was different about him—and what has distinguished him from so many others—is that he refused to accept the conventional scientific and social wisdom that said he must die.

This unknown person with limited personal funds decided not to surrender his life to the conventional wisdom or the lords of drug research. He would live. To do so, he would try anything and everything he could get his hands on. Not to subsist, but to really live. And, against all odds, he did. While opportunistic infections assailed his body, he underwent a stunning range of experimental therapies and endured.

He spent a year studying the disease. Using himself as a guinea pig and research laboratory, he became a lay expert on AIDS. He talked, asked questions, networked, and slowly came to understand how HIV works and how the human body functions under the unremitting assault of the disease.

At first, he just kept himself alive—barely. He was frequently very sick, often hospitalized. I wonder if he knows how he pulled through so many times. The process was slow and agonizing, physically and mentally. But the alternative was worse.

As a historian who has lost loved ones to AIDS, I became interested in Charles Caulfield and his story. I leave it to him to tell that story in his own way. What is important about him now—to all of us—is that he has seemingly done the impossible. He is not just a long-term survivor of AIDS. He has actually developed a workable plan of survival. A plan that works for him and is working for many others.

That is what this book is about. Not just how those infected with HIV can stay alive awhile longer, but how they can restore themselves. The plan, like the virus, changes, mutates. It is not set in stone. It is not the cure. But it is a beginning, a better beginning than all the resources of the National Institutes of Health.

Caulfield went on. He met Billi Goldberg, a treatment activist, and with her the plan was revised again and again, fine tuned. He became editor of "HIV News" in the San Francisco *Sentinel*, and his writings and ruminations struck a deep chord among readers everywhere. His work was copied and reprinted by admirers and vilified by the AIDS treatment establishment. He became controversial, a public figure of significant stature in what one activist ruefully calls "the world of AIDS."

Meanwhile, he and Goldberg went on challenging the conventional wisdom, the drug companies, and the establishment's fundamental approaches to AIDS. This unlikely pair of individuals began treating people with this plan, or with individually tailored components of it, and began to see results. Caulfield and Goldberg's findings were so extraordinary—while absolutely contrary to current scientific thinking—that the medical community could ignore them no longer. Several studies of their work are underway at major research centers. No one knows what the outcomes will be. But the benefits are already apparent: Now there is hope. Not hope for furthering the process of dying, but hope for at least partially restoring the immune functions of HIV-infected people.

Caulfield and Goldberg have done what billions of research dollars and the conventional medical establishment failed to do. Many years may pass before the HIV pandemic ends. But when the history of the fight against this disease is written, their places in it are assured.

James Blair Lovell
September, 1993
Washington, D.C.

Introduction

The *Anarchist AIDS Medical Formulary* is a collection of essays adapted from the San Francisco *Sentinel,* where they originally appeared in my regular column "HIV News." They are intended to guide the aspiring AIDS survivor into a new way of looking at AIDS, based on the most current, cutting-edge scientific discoveries in immunology.

When I first arrived in San Francisco in 1990, I was startled and dismayed at the lack of coordinated information on alternative medicine. What was available did not necessarily lend itself to validation by any accepted line of medical reasoning. I was appalled to find that many of the so-called "treatment advocacy" organizations had vested interests which compromised their ability to speak or act freely on behalf of people suffering from AIDS.

With my background in AIDS client advocacy and alternative treatment research, I felt a moral responsibility to step into this vacuum, and attempt to corroborate breakthroughs in science with promising therapies from the very active treatment underground. I never imagined the controversy which would ensue from embarking on this endeavor. I had unwittingly stepped into the eye of the storm.

The investigations I undertook, along with my research associate and kindred spirit, Ms. Billi Goldberg, are documented herein, chronicling the events in HIV treatment research for the one-year period between the 1992 Amsterdam and 1993 Berlin International Conferences on AIDS. They give a unique perspective into the inner machinations of society's response to this disease from the viewpoint of a medical reporter, himself diagnosed with AIDS, inside the maelstrom of the urban holocaust.

Much to my surprise, these essays as they first appeared in print gave way to a new dialogue on AIDS pathogenesis and treatment in both the local and national public health arenas. Polarizing the medical and activist communities into two opposing camps, the essays challenged outdated modes of thinking, and proposed new approaches to treatment. Ultimately, this work has resulted in profound changes in the research establishment's direction and orientation.

Most remarkably, this transformation was wholly initiated by two laypersons, without formal scientific training or significant financial resources. Through a rigorous, self-devised curriculum drawing from all branches of science, we achieved proficiency in the finer points of medicine, biochemistry, and immunology. The result of our enterprise has been an increasingly broad acceptance by scientists in government and academic research centers around the world. Our guerrilla immunology is now being integrated into the new medical paradigm emerging like the proverbial phoenix from the ashes of the medical establishment's failed response to the AIDS crisis. The entrenched competitiveness and baroque territoriality between various scientific disciplines has been the principal factor impeding progress in the development of effective strategies for medical intervention in HIV disease. Using the tenets of current basic science, we have been able to develop a strategy for immune reconstitution for people with AIDS. Our therapeutic system is nontoxic, effective, affordable, and readily available to all who need it.

It has been a long time since any real hope has been extended to people living with this disease. The *Anarchist AIDS Medical Formulary* delves deeply into revolutionary medical research and emerges bearing the "pearl of great price": a realistic therapeutic approach for survival and recovery from a disease which the majority of physicians still consider to be 100 percent fatal.

Throughout this anthology of essays, one connecting thread is always evident, and remains the basis of its message: AIDS is survivable. It is my intention that this work serve as a guide to finding the inner resources needed to surmount the challenge—as many of us have been able to do. Restoration of normal life expectancy with an extremely high quality of life for people with AIDS is now firmly within our reach. With courage and fortitude, anyone can avail themselves of the solution. We must however, grasp it with all our strength and stand strong against the harbingers of gloom.

By taking the leap into unknown territory, we find we have the momentum of the universe to assist us. An open mind, a willingness to learn, and a strong desire to live are all that are needed. Ten years after my diagnosis with an AIDS-defining illness, and my restoration to asymptomatic, immune competence, I can credibly state that this is not theory, but fact. I encourage you to join us in this adventure, as have many persons with AIDS who have been reconstituted to a state of immune competence and beaten the odds.

Part One

The Politics and Realities
of AIDS Treatment Research

Survival at Any Cost
(1/7/93)

Nine years ago to the day of this writing, I was on oxygen in the intensive care unit at the Medical Center of the University of California at San Diego. I had contracted what was then being called a "respiratory infection of unknown origin." A young Latino doctor, an infectious disease resident, walked into my room. Rather than approaching me, he stood and spoke to me from just inside the door. "We have a confirmed diagnosis from your sputum cultures, Mr. Caulfield." He was wearing a paper mask, so I was unable to detect any emotion on his part as he continued, "It's Pneumocystis carinii."

I didn't exactly know what that meant, but I could tell from the tone of his voice that it was nothing I wanted to hear. He didn't stick around after dropping the bomb. I was left alone in a deafening silence so clearly emblazoned in my memory it's as though it happened yesterday. I never saw that son of a bitch again. I received no further explanation from him. It was only later that a gay male nurse told me I had AIDS and explained the treatment: intravenous pentamidine intermittently for a week. They talked about removing my spleen. At that point, they didn't have a clue how to respond to the underlying disease or what caused it. They could only aggressively treat the pneumonia. I responded to the treatment and was released with a suggestion that I abstain from having sex.

The impression left on me by the heartless and fearful way I was handed a death sentence gave birth to my profound skepticism and mistrust of the American medical profession. This has undoubtedly been the primary reason that I remain relatively healthy compared to many people I know who have had the disease a much shorter time than I. Out of resentment, I looked for alternatives to what was seemingly inevitable at that time: death within a year, if I was lucky.

Since that time, with the help of many doctors along the way, I tried scores of underground AIDS treatments. AZT was not to come

3

for another three and a half years. *Any* treatment at that point was "alternative," the only alternative to death. I decided to go for it.

In the ensuing years, I crossed paths with many other PWAs who had decided to do whatever it took to fight for their lives. We shared and compared information, and a true "underground railroad" of alternative treatment began to emerge. From Tijuana, Mexico, people were bringing in two drugs, Ribavirin, an antiviral, and Isoprinosine, an alleged immune stimulant. You could get them from some groups of buyers, but no one was sure how to use them in correct dosages. There are PWAs today who believe that those two substances kept them alive until something better came along. At the same time, through the work of Project Inform, the U.S. government relaxed its restrictions on the illegal importation of therapeutic agents. Some "crazy" doctors were getting together and comparing notes on potential treatments. A movement was gaining momentum. People were taking risks and some lived to tell about them.

A recipe for making a home mixture of egg lipids (AL–721) based on research in Israel was widely circulated. An anti-atherosclerosis drug (Dextran Sulfate) from Japan was being imported as an antiviral. Extracts from mistletoe, aloe vera, and pine cones were imported illegally from Germany and Switzerland. It was reported that people were painting a photographic industry chemical (DNCB) on their skin to stimulate their immune systems. John James in *Aids Treatment News* began chronicling reported developments and options and how to obtain the treatments. Tom O'Connor published his book *Living With AIDS,*[1] which gave in minute detail the then current "possibly helpful" treatment options drawn from nutrition, macrobiotics, herbal medicine, and Western pharmacology. Buyers' clubs emerged and thrived.

Over the years, by trial and error, I arrived at combinations of treatments which worked to a greater or lesser extent for various periods of time. Most were worthless. Some seemed to help for a little while and then their effectiveness dropped off. A precious few, when used in certain combinations, seemed to push the disease into remission for long periods of time.

It would be an exercise in futility to state categorically what treatment strategy I use, since no one thing works for everybody. I believe that enough information is available so that everybody can find treatments they can afford. Finding the will and inner strength to take on the healing process is the challenge of every aspiring AIDS survivor.

I have no survivor's guilt. I'm not one of the "lucky" ones. I worked my ass off educating myself, trying new treatments, and growing. I selected from what I thought was useful from my doctor and many other sources. AZT was never an option; I tried it briefly in 1987 and was not able to tolerate it.

I am quite certain that it's no accident I have lived this long. My willingness to keep my eyes and mind open, to discover and do whatever was needed to survive, opened doors of opportunity that I would never have believed possible. Bizarre coincidences and chance meetings were common along the way.

Most people who were diagnosed the same year as I died within six to twelve months. Yet, I personally know scores of people who, like myself, remain healthy and well after living through a host of ungodly opportunistic illnesses. We're still exchanging information, comparing notes, and pushing for changes in the service delivery system. Having seen so many people die makes me angry enough to keep researching and publishing my notes from the underground guerrilla clinics. The information I relay must be about therapies that people can readily obtain and afford. Otherwise, what good is it? Nothing is worse than reading about a clinical trial of a potentially useful drug and then not meeting the eligibility criteria, or hearing of a new treatment that is prohibitively expensive. Just as in the beginning of the AIDS epidemic, people need nontoxic treatments and they need them now! They need effective, affordable treatments that they can research and start on right away, and that won't kill them. And most importantly, people living with AIDS need accurate information on options they are not likely to hear about from their doctors.

I believe in the value of conventional Western medicine, but thus far, it has not offered a viable solution to AIDS. A candid, ongoing exchange among PWAs outside the influence of the "nonprofit" agencies is critical to our survival. Since we bear most directly the consequences of how research dollars are spent, we must have critical input into how decisions are made.

Nine years ago, I would never have believed that I would live even half as long as I have. I'm now thirty-seven and have been diagnosed with AIDS for a quarter of my lifetime. However long I have actually been infected with HIV, only God knows. My moment of truth came in that hospital room in January, 1984, when I felt just angry enough to begin to question everything. I ruthlessly gathered information, made treatment choices that felt right for me, and passed the information along. This process has served me well. I'm counting on being around for a while and taking another look back.

Acceptable Risks by Jonathan Kwitny
(9/24/92)

Jonathan Kwitny's *Acceptable Risks* might better be titled, "Indiana Jones and the FDA."[2] The cover blurb describes it as "the explosive politics of life vs. profit in America—How two courageous men fought the FDA To save thousands of AIDS patients and changed the drug industry forever." The story of Martin Delaney and Jim Corti, as told to a *Wall Street Journal* feature writer, reads like an election year "authorized biography," heavy on ideology, soft on content. This might be forgivable, though, in light of the fact that its subjects are not likely to be treated so kindly by history.

Acceptable Risks presents a sweeping chronology of Project Inform's highjinks with the National Cancer Institute's Sam Broder and the development of an underground AIDS drug-running operation into a federally-funded pharmaceutical industry political action committee. The heroes of the story are cast as an unlikely combination of James Bond and Mother Theresa.

According to the book, these two brave men, with never a thought for themselves, and with the acquiescence of the treatment underground, developed protocols for treatments using Ribavirin, Isoprinosine, Dextran Sulphate, and Compound Q, all in order to save desperate AIDS patients. Their combative, forceful lobbying at the National Institute of Allergy and Infectious Diseases (NIAID) and the Food and Drug Administration (FDA) pressed into place a medical ideology in which dissent has been rendered heretical. Their ability to manipulate a chaotic national public health response into the molding hands of powerful pharmaceutical industry giants is a wonder to behold. The story of how the nefarious nonprofit fund-awarding policies of these drug companies allowed Project Inform to become what is perceived as the credible voice of treatment advocacy is undeniably without parallel in FDA history.

Yet a vague unfamiliarity arises in the reader. Memory is haunted by the strange recollection that there was more to the saga than is revealed in the pages of this dramatic thriller. What this book fails to recount warrants serious consideration of just what Project Inform's founders would like us to forget. Specifically, a few glaring omissions from this tailored retelling seem rather odd to this reviewer.

First, there's hardly a mention of AL–721, which, prior to the marketing of AZT, was the underground treatment of choice for people with AIDS. This substance generated enormous dialogue involving Martin Delaney and the FDA, and was reported by the "venerable" *AIDS Treatment News* on numerous occasions as "appearing to work." AL–721, a nontoxic, affordable, and possibly effective treatment for AIDS, was completely discarded by the mainstream and the underground after a single tiny, loosely-controlled clinical trial at St. Luke's/Roosevelt Hospital in New York. Then, for some strange reason, the researchers hurriedly bestowed favor on a class of drugs with then unknown potential for toxicity and a price tag that stunned Wall Street and AIDS activists equally. Despite the fact that the book purports to tell us that these two swashbuckling advocates of the dying were busily working to change the drug industry forever, it doesn't seem to have room in its 400-plus pages for a brief mention of such a "trifling event."

Acceptable Risks also neglects to mention the uncomfortable little matter of the Dextran Sulphate side effects problem. Dextran Sulphate, a complex sugar molecule used in Japan to treat atherosclerosis, showed promise in the test tube as a substance that would synergize the effects of AZT, thus allowing for lower, presumably less toxic doses of the drug. The drug running-cabal, once more advocating selflessly for the desperate, failed to notify its constituents that physicians in clinical practice were observing severe side effects, such as gastrointestinal bleeding, since Dextran Sulphate breaks down in the system into sulphuric acid. Of course, our "heroes" did eventually become a bit less enthusiastic about the drug, but issued no warnings until the already imported stock of the drug had been dispensed.

Maybe mainstream America will be enamored by this work of historical fiction. Those who lived in urban Gay America during the period described by *Acceptable Risks* should approach this little piece of public relations with caution. The gay community's memory seems sometimes to falter in matters of those posing as our friends and advocates. Through forwarding what it claims to be "our" agenda, Project Inform has become the federally recognized voice for the medical needs of PWAs. In a year in which San Francisco's AIDS budget is being shredded, Project Inform is doing just fine. Receiving corporate donations from the drug companies and federal funds through Ryan White CARE allocations, they have become an integral part of the bureaucracy they arose to combat. Throughout the book, Delaney repeatedly states that the drugs worked fine, it was the bureaucracy that was intransigent. Delaney may find that the bureaucracy now works the way he wants it to. Unfortunately for us, the drugs themselves leave much to be desired.

If you are interested in finding out what is really going on in AIDS treatment, I suggest you take the twenty-four dollar retail cost of this book, and take a PWA out to dinner. Ask him or her, and you'll most likely be told that the pain and demoralization endured through their medical history is not a bit assuaged by this piece of self-aggrandizement for which each copy sold will place money in the pockets of these two self-styled "heroes" of the AIDS epidemic.

New Controversy over HIV and Suntanning (11/12/92)

On September 21, 1992, a complaint was filed with the California State Board of Medical Examiners against Marcus Conant, M.D., a clinical professor of Dermatology at University of California at San Francisco, and director of what he calls the "largest private AIDS clinic in the world." The complaint, filed by San Francisco DNCB treatment activist Billi Goldberg, alleges that Conant recommends immune suppressive therapies for dermatological manifestations of HIV disease, such as psoriasis and a disorder known as eosinophilic folliculitis. Goldberg maintains that Conant compromises long-term health for superficial short-term results. The issue revolves around Conant's recommendation that his HIV patients experiencing excessive discomfort caused by psoriasis may gain some relief from exposure to ultraviolet (UV) light. This contradicts the generally held belief that UV radiation harms the immune system.

Dr. Conant kindly agreed to speak with me in a recent interview to respond to the charge. He answered Goldberg's complaint with this statement: "I have recommended controlled exposure to ultraviolet light, stressing to the patient that he or she should be certain that they tan only without obtaining enough UV light to burn."[3] An article in a recent issue of the highly respected journal *Science* states that "a significant proportion of HIV-infected individuals have dermatological conditions that may be candidates for PUVA (psoralen ultraviolet-A light) therapy, which could do more harm than good if it really activates latent HIV in the Langerhan cells of the skin."[4] The article also reported that most researchers in the field believe that a side effect of the DNA damage caused by UV type-A radiation is the activation of HIV expression. In a letter responding to the *Science* article, National Cancer Institute researchers Mario Clerici and Gene Shearer support the danger of UV exposure, stating that "UV exposure could also excacerbate progression to AIDS by interfering with protective immunity."[5]

During our discussion, Conant stated that in situations in which the patient's quality of life is so severely impaired by problems related to AIDS psoriasis, and other treatments are not an option—due to the even more immunosuppressive side effects of other conventional therapies—he would not advise against moderate exposure to sunlight (which contains both UV–A and UV–B light waves) to obtain some degree of symptom relief.

Goldberg has countered this with a reference to Conant's own article "Future Issues in AIDS" published in the journal *Dermatologic Clinics.*[6] In the same issue, leading dermatology authority Madelaine Duvic stated that "in vitro studies show that ultraviolet light activates

HIV gene expression, and we have seen patients develop Kaposi's Sarcoma while receiving ultraviolet irradiation."[7]

Conant stressed that he was certain to caution his patients of the danger of burning, but experts do not agree as to the volume of exposure to UV–A light needed to activate dormant HIV. He added that he would make such a recommendation only after soberly weighing the risks of exposure against the quality of life impairment caused by the skin problems themselves. Other treatments for HIV psoriasis include high dosages of AZT (1200 to 1500 mg. per day), and topical steroid drugs, both of which have their own immunosuppressive side effects. "Physicians are really in a quandary regarding this matter," Conant said. "It is difficult for us to draw the line where quality of life is so inhibited that long-term risks can be assumed in order to obtain immediate symptom relief."

In a recent issue of the San Francisco-based *AIDS Treatment News*,[8] John S. James reported on current research demonstrating that people with HIV are strikingly unaware of this risk, and were three times more likely to use a sunbed regularly than HIV-negative individuals, in the belief that a suntan would improve their health. The high numbers of tanning salons in the Castro and other popular gay neighborhoods in San Francisco highlight the degree to which the gay community is targeted by the tanning industry. HIV-positive people must be aware of the broad medical consensus that HIV's destruction of the immune system may be accelerated by exposure to ultraviolet light in tanning salons. James concluded that "it is important to warn the community, even while we wait for definitive information. Nobody knows why HIV disease progresses much faster in some people than in others. If ultraviolet light, among other factors, contributes to faster disease progression, it probably would have escaped notice."

Caulfield Responds to Physician's Rebuttal
(11/19/92)

My article "New Controversy Over HIV and Suntanning" drew a significant number of responses from readers. Among these, a San Francisco physician's response underplayed the significance of the risk of HIV viral activation by moderate exposure to UV radiation through the use of tanning beds and exposure to sunlight.

However, contrary to this physician's assertion that "virtually all tanning beds in current use are claimed to emit pure UVA radiation," independent research, including an interview with an electronics specialist affiliated with Sun-Days Tanning Centers, led me to a different conclusion. I found that contrary to the doctor's statement, both UVA and UVB radiation are commonly used in the tanning beds that are a mainstay of the industry. Specialized tanning beds which emit only type-A radiation, where available, cost four times as much of the more common tanning beds utilizing both UVA and UVB.

In all fairness to the distinguished physician's rebuttal, a thorough review of the medical literature discussing the effect of ultraviolet radiation on the immune response revealed a number of errors in his statements. His suggestion that UV–A radiation "only slightly" acts in a manner which could activate HIV expression is in stark contrast to an article in the *International Journal of Dermatology,* in which two dermatologists from the University of San Diego School of Medicine state that "Ultraviolet A is capable of causing various types of structural damage to DNA. It is conceivable that reduction of Langerhans cells by UVA radiation results in inefficient immunodestruction of early neoplastic cells . . . allowing the exposure to be expressed in the form of tumors."[9] The *Science* article I cited previously asserts that UVA radiation is a necessary prerequisite for the awakening of HIV from dormancy.

I must also question my respondent's allegation that UV type-C radiation is the constituent in sunlight most dangerous for the immune system. This is clearly contradicted in the text *Immune Mechanisms in Cutaneous Disease.* The authors state, "UVC is potentially the most harmful of the ultraviolet radiations. Fortunately, UVC does not reach the earth's surface because it is effectively absorbed by the ozone in the upper atmosphere."[10]

In his letter, the physician admitted to advising his patients that nonburning exposure to sunlight is "all right, but a good number eight sunscreen is necessary." Yet, again according to the *International Journal of Dermatology* article, many sunscreen formulations claim UVA protection, but in fact none of them block all UVA rays. A clear link appears to exist between exposure to UVA and UVB radiation and immunosuppressive effects on subcutaneous Langerhans cells impairing their ability to signal the proliferation of CD4 cells.[11] It may also cause cellular DNA damage resulting in acceleration of viral expression. The danger is clearly stated in current medical peer review journals.[12]

In keeping with previous warnings[13] and published medical research, the HIV community should take note of the potential danger of exposure to sunlight and tanning beds. Their potential for immune suppression and viral activation may play a key role in accelerating the decline and death of people living with HIV.[14]

1992 and the Emergence of the New Activism (12/31/92)

Paul Volberding and Donald Abrams, two of the most reputable leaders in the AIDS medical community, admitted this year for the first time the futility of the current regime of antiviral treatments for HIV. Both physicians, pioneers in antiviral drug therapy for HIV, wrote in editorials published in the *Bulletin of Experimental Treatments for AIDS* that while the currently used drug therapies AZT, ddI, and ddC may show a transient increase in CD4s, they do not extend survival time, but merely delay the onset of symptoms.[15] Abrams quoted a study in which the authors state that the effects of early therapy on survival and the optimal time to initiate therapy remain controversial even for AZT, the cornerstone of antiretroviral therapy.[16] In his editorial, Abrams lamented, "But we really must face the critical issue and not pooh-pooh survival in favor of modest transient increases in CD4 counts, or even significantly decreased short-term disease progression." Abrams states what few doctors dare to admit publicly: "The ultimate progression of HIV disease, unfortunately, continues to be towards death as an endpoint." This despite the billions spent on drug research.

The Eighth International Conference on AIDS in Amsterdam on July 19–24, 1992, clearly demonstrated that new therapies previously thought promising have shown no efficacy, with no meaningful new antiviral treatments in development. One of the most noteworthy events of the Conference was the presentation of the single didactic module on alternative treatments, highlighting nutrition, Chinese Medicine, DNCB, and other potential treatments from outside the mainstream.

This year also saw the virtual collapse of Project Inform, cheerleader and pimp for the drug industry's toxic "drug of the week" marketing strategy. And, down from what was once a grass-roots organization of hundreds of effective activists, ACT-UP Golden Gate's membership has been reduced to approximately thirty.

But perhaps 1992's most notable development is the growth of a highly evolved meta-network of computer bulletin boards, created by individuals tracing alternative sources to call attention to the discrepancies between theory and practice. The establishment's failure to find an effective therapy for this disease has largely been a by-product of institutional territoriality between virologists, molecular biologists, and oncologists. University researchers, fiercely guarding their own agendas and research dollars, have failed to discuss the obvious failure of conventional therapies.

However, some clinicians and scientists, who see all too clearly the futility of the mainstream treatment options, have joined the efforts of the electronic watchdogs. The evolution of such a complex system of instantaneous communication has fomented a worldwide dialogue that now has begun to drive the AIDS treatment development agenda. This global exchange makes full use of cutting-edge research in immunology and other relevant disciplines working in the design of AIDS treatments. The online bulletin board system now allows specialists to share information and learn from other clinicians, the patients themselves, and the new "lay learned"—individuals who, dissatisfied with the chronic lack of progress, have taken it upon themselves to learn the basic science and engage credibly in the ongoing dialogue on AIDS therapies.

International computer bulletin boards facilitate discussion between scientists and activists in Europe, South America, the United Kindgom, Africa, and throughout the United States. One such service, HIV/AIDS Info BBS, is operated by Sister Mary Elizabeth, a nun in the order of the Sisters of Elizabeth of Hungary in San Juan Capistrano, California. Their online bulletin board makes available the texts of all primary AIDS publications, abstracts of medical journal references on AIDS, FDA reports, and the Centers for Disease Control daily summaries. HIV/AIDS Info BBS also hosts the AEGIS (AIDS Education General Information Service) Network. Online conferences sponsored by AEGIS include AIDS.DIALOGUE, AIDS.DATA, AIDS.DRUGS, AIDS.SPIRITUAL, AIDS.TRIALS, and AIDS.WOMEN, all of which are exported all over the world. Linking with HIVNET in Amsterdam and GreenNet in London, AEGIS has evolved into a true global electronic network for AIDS. *See Resource Guide, p. 153.*

Fidonet International AIDS/ARC, AIDS-HIV, and USENET sci.med.aids and bionet.molbio.hiv, are all international vehicles for interactive dialogue on subjects pertaining to AIDS treatment. Membership in San Francisco's International Global Communications allows access to USENET sci.med.aids and E-mail for a nominal fee. All other bulletin board services mentioned here offer membership free of charge, with access to posting and receiving questions, answers, and hypotheses.

Rather than waiting for the lengthy process of medical journal publication, professionals now have available instantaneous peer review of their theories and treatment regimens by tens of thousands of interdisciplinary practitioners, as well as by knowledgeable PWAs. This rapid exchange of important information stands in stark contrast to what was previously available to treatment advocates, who had to rely on time-consuming and expensive "snail-mail." Material sent by conventional means is very possibly outdated by the time it is received by the subscriber. One exception is *AIDS Treatment News,* which has always freely and readily allowed computer bulletin board access.

Many scientists, doctors, and researchers are surprisingly computer illiterate, and, unable to utilize this method of rapid communication, are being left behind. Computer-savvy activists gain a pronounced advantage in acquiring the most up-to-date information, as well as the dialogue needed to make sense of it. Institutional and disciplinary boundaries are being circumvented in the development of this information exchange network. This allows for the free exchange of information so vital to the search for an AIDS cure.

Looking back at 1992, it is apparent that *The Sentinel* has courageously gone beyond the middle-of-the-road stance of most of the popular gay press. Many alternative theories on the origin and treatment of AIDS have been aired in these pages. In the coming year, I will continue to offer thoroughly researched, credible data with which to make informed treatment choices.

Happy New Year. May 1993 be the Year of the Cure.

Cytotoxic T-Cells and Disease Progression in AIDS (1/21/93)

CD4 T-lymphocytes have long been considered the most significant markers of disease progression in AIDS. When their number declines, the onset of opportunistic infections is predictable. A breakthrough in AIDS research came when CD4 T-cell numbers were substituted for death in clinical trials, gaining them the dubious title of "surrogate markers."

Recent state-of-the-art research indicates that CD8 T-cells, also known as cytotoxic lymphocytes, play a crucial role in determining the patient's immune status. Despite this, many physicians in clinical practice are reticent to abandon outdated measurements of disease progression in AIDS. Currently the most widely used laboratory predictors of disease progression are p24 antigen and antibody tests, beta-2 microglobulin, CD4 counts, and neopterin levels, all of which are drawn from blood tests. Yet the medical community clearly recognizes that the majority of viral infections and pathogens which are opportunistic in AIDS reside primarily in the mucous membranes of the body. Blood laboratory evidence is therefore of questionable value.

The importance in maintaining CD8 counts is only now being widely recognized in AIDS treatment. Two submissions for presentations at next year's Ninth International Conference on AIDS in Berlin, drawn from research in two entirely different fields of study, close with statements to the effect that halting of disease progression is associated over periods of time with stable CD8 counts.[17] This is despite possible declines, in some cases to zero, in CD4 counts.

Both papers speculate that stable CD8 counts may be a common denominator in long-term survival, as Dr. Jay Levy of University of California at San Francisco has long asserted. But patients seldom ask about their CD8 counts, and physicians seldom volunteer the information. With this information, a patient might consider a therapy aimed at increasing and stabilizing these critical cells.

Several approaches to increasing CD8s in symptomatic individuals are under investigation. A pilot Kaposi's Sarcoma (KS) treatment called CD8 Cell Expansion, in which CD8 T-cells are removed from the blood and cultivated in culture by adding the protein Interleukin-2, is currently fully enrolled and underway in San Francisco. Another method increasing CD8 T-cells is to modify the body's biological response. Topical application of DNCB has been consistently shown to nontoxically raise CD8 counts and natural killer cells among compliant patients. With such results, DNCB is understandably receiving increasing attention among patients and physicians around the world.

What we need are accurate measurements of viral replication in mucosal tissue and in the lymphatic system, where the greatest populations of virus and other pathogens reside. The science already exists, in what is known as polymerase technology. A laboratory test called the Reverse Transcriptase Polymerase Chain Reaction (RT-PCR) is the "gold standard" for determining the activity of tissue virus. RT-PCR therefore has incomparable value in assessing the effectiveness of drugs intended to interfere with viral replication. In addition, a subset of T-lymphocytes known as CD38s, immature CD8s, have been shown to correspondingly increase with a patient's clinical decline.

Why are these laboratory tests not in everyday use, even at leading Medical Centers? Many researchers, scientists, and activists realize that this is one of the most critical issues in turning around twelve years of bungling and getting on the right track toward finding effective treatments quickly. Of course, it is certain that pharmaceutical industry profiteers will not take too kindly to any revision of the status quo, even if it does result from current discoveries in immunology.

Our morbid preoccupation with certain "magic" numbers in CD4 counts was fostered back in 1987, when Burroughs Wellcome set 200 CD4s as the required T-cell decline to qualify for AZT. Most current antiviral therapies for HIV use blood tests to evaluate their effectiveness, yet, as I mentioned previously, the substantial viral load is not in the bloodstream. It would seem that certain organizations and institutions have a vested interest in disregarding the newest data, and use their enormous influence to ensure that many others remain clueless, as well. In this perverse game of life vs. profit, guess who wins?

Present Focus of AIDS Research Is Wrong
(1/21/93)
Billi Goldberg

On January 5, 1993, the *New York Times* published an article by AIDS writer Gina Kolata on new research questioning various theories that HIV is not involved in AIDS.[18] Kolata stated, "Researchers have found that more human cells are actually latently infected with HIV, which helps explain how the entire immune system is eventually destroyed. In 1986, it was believed that only one in 1,000 white blood cells were infected with the virus. But now, researchers are finding that 10, 20, even 30 percent of white blood cells may carry HIV, in addition to other cells. As a result, researchers conclude that direct infection with HIV should be sufficient to explain the destruction of the immune system in AIDS patients." This research was recently reported in the *Proceedings of the National Academy of Sciences.*[19]

For a decade, the goal driving HIV/AIDS research has been to increase peripheral blood CD4 counts. In clinical trials, CD4 counts were the primary "surrogate markers" used to ascertain efficacy of the test drugs. Approved treatments have suppressed the immune system's ability to destroy infected CD4 cells, resulting in transient increases in their numbers. Considering that there are many people still alive with no peripheral blood CD4 cells and many people who have died with CD4 counts in the hundreds, it is obvious that this approach is at best mistaken, and deliberately false, at worst.

Viral and most opportunistic infections in AIDS are intracellular. Intracellular and extracellular pathogens have different means of expressing their presence. One researcher has stated, "This has led to the interpretation that CD8 and CD4 T-cells have a division of tasks:

CD8 CTLs control intracellular pathogens whereas CD4 helper T-cells help to eradicate extracellular pathogens by cooperation with B-cells and by release of cytokines."[20]

D. F. Nixon, a molecular immunologist, states in the book *Immunology of Infection* that "The normal immune response to an infectious organism involves both nonspecific and antigen-specific immunity. Virus infections stimulate specific antibodies, T-helper cells and cytotoxic T-cells (CTL). The importance of virus-specific CTL in the clearance of viral infections has been increasingly recognized over the past decade, and it is likely that CTL form the major specific defence against primary virus infections."[21]

These facts raise a serious question: Has all the HIV/AIDS treatment research for the past ten years been wrong? Since there is little doubt that from 10 to 30 percent or more of tissue CD4 cells are infected, increasing their number would serve to increase the number of infected CD4 cells. Research has shown that AZT suppresses the immune response, significantly affecting proliferating CD8 cytotoxic lymphocytes.[22] It is natural for the immune system to destroy infected self-cells such as CD4. Inhibiting the process can only result in uncontrolled replication of HIV.

The focus on AIDS research must shift to stimulating, activating, and increasing the CD8 and other cytotoxic lymphocytes in the immune system, disregarding the CD4 cells.[23] Since it is the evolutionary responsibility of the cytotoxic T-lymphocytes to destroy infected and abnormal self-cells, increasing their numbers would be beneficial. A treatment strategy concentrating on boosting the HIV/AIDS weakened immune system with biological response modifiers (BRM), that act specifically on cytotoxic CD8 cells and other lymphocyte killer cells, then becomes the obvious path.

Fauci Says HIV Latency Period "A Myth"
(2/11/93)

In the February 4, 1992 edition of the prestigious *New England Journal of Medicine,* researchers Anthony Fauci and associates from the Laboratory of Immune Regulation, National Institute for Allergies and Infectious Diseases, published their thesis "The Immunopatho-genesis of HIV Infection."[24] The paper, in clear terms, dispels several widely-held myths about AIDS in conventional medicine.

In an important passage, Fauci states that "although the clinical course [of HIV infection] is characterized by a prolonged period of latency after primary infection, HIV replication continues at high lev-els in the lymphoid organs during this period." It is commonly, albeit incorrectly, believed that HIV remains dormant for up to ten years before initiating immune damage. Fauci's findings indicate that much of the damage done to the immune system occurs during what appears to be the "asymptomatic" stage.

Fauci disputes the efficacy of blood measurements of disease pro-gression with the statement, "peripheral blood measurements do not accurately reflect the total body burden of HIV infection; the lym-phoid organs are the major reservoirs of virus and sites of viral repli-cation." This indicates that Fauci believes that measurements of p24 antigen, neopterin levels, and CD4 counts from blood are useless as predictive markers, since the blood does not harbor the majority of the body's viral load.

Fauci avers that by the time of the onset of symptoms, the lym-phoid organs will have become massive generators of the vectors of disease. He adds, "The term 'clinical latency' is misleading, how-ever, since during this period virtually all patients have a gradual deterioration of the immune system, manifested particularly through the depletion of CD4 T-cells.... Hence, in certain pathologic processes involving lymphoid cells, the peripheral blood may not accurately reflect the status of disease. Furthermore, specific immune responses are generated predominantly in the lymphoid organs rather than in the peripheral blood." Fauci goes on to say that less than 2 percent of the body's lymphocytes, or T-cells, exist in the blood; the remaining 98 percent reside in the mucosal tissues and lymphoid organs.

I have frequently stated in "HIV News" that state-of-the-art tech-nology is needed to in measure viral load and activity in the lymph nodes and mucosa. These measurements should be given precedence over CD4 measurements which newer technology has rendered prac-tically useless. Fauci's article reiterates the importance of widespread use of the polymerase technology that measures total body viral load. Blood measurements such as p24, neopterin, and CD4 cell counts are increasingly useless. At present, polymerase technology is expensive, costing hundreds of dollars, but so were CD4 counts just a few years ago. As the technology has become commonplace, a CD4 count can now be obtained for less than thirty dollars. As it comes into wider use, the Polymerase Chain Reaction Assay will become an invaluable diagnostic tool. Accordingly, its cost will decrease. Fauci's paper, as well as the evolving positions of researchers from all over the world, continue to drive home the fact that the current focus of AIDS treatment research is fatally flawed.

Abrams Presents Contradictory Views on Antivirals (3/4/93)

In spite of several recently published essays on the inability of nucleoside analogue drugs to prolong survival in the patients who use them, San Francisco General Hospital's Donald Abrams, M.D., gave a half-hearted recounting of studies comparing ddI, ddC, and AZT at a recent Community Forum.[25] In his colorless presentation, entitled "Strategies of Antiviral Therapies," Abrams' only commentary on the state of antiviral treatments for HIV was that ddI, ddC, and AZT appeared to be more similar in effect than previously thought.

Yet Abrams' editorial, "On the Matter of Survival," published in the November, 1992 edition of the *Bulletin of Experimental Treatments for AIDS,* contained a statement that some have interpreted as a sign of his disillusionment: "It is certainly difficult, and a bit unsettling, to face uncertainties that still remain in the field of treatment of HIV. . . . But we really must face the critical issue and not pooh-pooh survival in favor of modest transient increases in CD4, or even significantly decreased short-term disease progression." Abrams asserts that differences between AZT, ddI, and ddC are virtually negligible, and further, that none of the drugs in any combination extended the life expectancy of the patient.

Abrams further elaborated on his concerns about earlier intervention with antiretroviral therapies in another recent article, replete with such scary quotes as: "Some may argue that this is the best way to treat infectious disease—early utilization of effective agents. Is enough really known to make such a recommendation in HIV disease?"[26] Such public ambivalence, coupled with Abrams' willingness to prescribe early therapy with nucleosides, indicates an unconscionable duplicity.

Dr. Abrams has repeatedly made abysmal assessments of the use of antiretroviral therapy in print. Yet, he appears as the guest speaker at the Conant Foundation's monthly presentation neutrally presenting data that suggests that AZT, ddI, and ddC are equally ineffective in prolonging survival time. This physician, who played a crucial role in the adoption of this line of chemical treatment, now seems discouraged and cynical. In the meantime, these "therapeutic agents" known to be responsible for significant organ and bone marrow toxicity, with marginal, if any, therapeutic benefit, have become the mainstays of HIV antiretroviral therapy. In presenting this information scientifically, without divulging his true opinion which diverges starkly from the material he presented, Abrams gave one of the most hypocritical stage performances of a public health presentation seen to date in San Francisco.

Drs. Abrams and Conant disregarded questions about Fauci's article in the *New England Journal of Medicine,* in which it was clearly stated that blood measurement of immune parameters misrepresents total body viral burden and fails to register immune reactions specific to the lymphatic organs were disregarded.[27] The question of diagnostic techniques is critical to the evaluation of drug effectiveness. As Fauci's and other labs have demonstrated, the germinal centers of the lymph nodes are the breeding ground for the majority of the body's viral burden. When asked how it is determined whether the currently used antiviral drugs are able to reach and inhibit viral replication at these germinal centers, neither Dr. Abrams nor Dr. Conant were able to respond to the question. Asked to comment on treatments he had helped pioneer, such as DNCB, Abrams stated that he had seen remarkable health and longevity in DNCB users, although these were isolated cases.

At no point during the presentation was there any discussion of the human element of treatment. Abrams instead relied heavily on charts and statistical didactic material. His lackluster presentation apparently belied a jaded and pessimistic outlook on the current state of antivirals.

As I have stated repeatedly in "HIV News," a new direction in treatment research is imperative—one utilizing the body's own complex biological interactions to compensate for the lymphatic organs damage, increase cellular presentation of antigens, and elicit cytotoxic destruction of infected cells. Unfortunately, the focus of the recent Community Forum continued to inexorably dwell on futile attempts to "kill the virus" with antivirals. It's time to admit the obvious: nucleoside drugs do more harm than good with the long-term immune suppression they engender.

Stimulating the immune system's innate ability to generate populations of cytotoxic T-lymphocytes which identify and eliminate cells infected with all intracellular pathogens, including viruses, will make AIDS a livable disease. But until the clinicians are able to admit the failure of their previous course of treatment, no progress can be made. This discrepancy between theory and practice, especially in the area of diagnosis, must be eliminated.

Zip Code Genocide
(3/11/93)

A few weeks ago, the National Research Council produced a document entitled "The Social Impact of AIDS," in which the AIDS epidemic is reduced to a minor sociological phenomenon primarily limited to minority populations in specific urban areas.[28] The Council document states that AIDS "is settling into spatially and socially isolated groups," while "many geographic areas and strata of the population are virtually untouched by the epidemic and probably never will be."

Council spokesman Dr. Don C. Des Jarlais was quoted in the *New York Times* saying, "We could stamp out AIDS without a vaccine or even a wonder drug."[29] Jarlais, a drug abuse specialist at New York's Beth Israel Hospital and a member of the National AIDS Commission, went on to describe the Research Council's ominous plan.

Council member and State University of New York Sociologist Dr. John Gagnon reportedly said, "We've got to put the money where the problem is." He proposes concentrating the "War on AIDS" to twenty-three or thirty neighborhoods in San Francisco, Houston, New York, Miami, and other cities. Studies previously conducted in New York City showed that the epidemic clustered in less than a dozen specific neighborhoods. According to Council member Dr. James Trussell, director of the Office of Population Research at Princeton, disease occurrence could be further sequestered epidemiologically, identifying six to ten New York neighborhoods in which HIV infection clustered in two of nine zip codes. Trussell was reported to have said that "If we had done case studies in other cities in the depth that we did in New York City, we would find the same thing."

In its assessment of the long-term sociological effects of the epidemic, this report minimizes the cost in lives due to AIDS. It states that with the passage of time, the AIDS epidemic will become little more than a footnote in the "warp and woof of historical events." The report predicts a future bearing few scars from the era of AIDS. It is safe to assume that the membership of the National Research Council neither belong to the culturally specific groups it has identified, nor live in the delineated geographic areas in which this disease "occurs."

In the last few years, much progress has been made in AIDS education, helping to lessen discrimination against groups severely affected by the epidemic. This was accomplished largely by shifting the focus from "high risk groups" to "high risk behaviors." The Council report proposes a radically redirected approach, targeting narrow segments of society for prevention measures. The result of this shift of emphasis is a backward step towards increased discrimination against gays, blacks, IV drug users, and other groups targeted as "carriers" of the disease and threats to society.

Identifying certain groups, whether infected or not, through such artificial means as zip code distribution, will likely lead to serious consequences—decreased property values, rejection of insurance coverage, higher rates of unemployment, and other forms of social and economic ostracism. In cities less progressive than San Francisco, targeted groups may find their neighborhoods increasingly "ghettoized" and isolated from the larger community.

An Orwellian scenario is easy to imagine: "carriers" will be allowed, perhaps assisted, to die, in order to erase the threat of AIDS to the "general population." Is this the true method being proposed by these eminent researchers, who apparently feel somehow magically insulated from the reach of this disease? If their families and other loved ones were to become members of these culturally and geographically isolated groups, the Council members might find that AIDS is not so casually relegated to a "historical footnote."

The Council report places little emphasis on the number of carrier deaths required to "stamp out AIDS." Even at the embarrassingly conservative perennial government estimate of one million infected individuals in the United States, the loss of life would be horrific. "The Social Impact of AIDS" is nothing more than a modern-day Wannsee Conference proposing a racist, homophobic segregationism. The dangerous ideas it proposes hold the potential for a Warsaw ghetto-like existence for PWAs, and virtual genocide before all infected individuals cease to pose a public health threat. Only then will the National Research Council be able to write their "historical footnote."

Prominent AIDS Researcher
Makes Bleak Predictions
(3/18/93)

William A. Haseltine, a prominent AIDS Researcher at the Dana Farber Cancer Institute in Boston and a frequent consultant to the NIH, recently made a series of grim predictions about the future of AIDS. These predictions include AIDS infection of forty to 100 million people worldwide by the year 2000; by the year 2025, as many as one billion people will be infected with the human immunodeficiency virus.

Drawing on data from studies conducted jointly by the World Health Organization and Harvard University, Haseltine presented a dark vision of the future at the annual meeting of the American Association for the Advancement of Science held recently in Boston. In his address, Haseltine said, "Projecting that 20 percent of major world populations will be infected with HIV is not unreasonable."[30]

Haseltine cited little known statistics on worldwide epidemiology. In Thailand, 20 percent of all young men entering the army are HIV-positive; the government of India is projecting that 10 percent of all adults in many urban areas will be infected by the year 2005. Haseltine noted that the United States, the Western nation with the highest incidence of HIV infection, has never conducted a broad, systematic study of blood samples to determine how many people have been exposed to HIV.

The U.S. Public Health Service has reported an estimated one million cases of infection in Americans every year since 1986. Haseltine's data implies this statistic is unfounded by any scientifically recognized surveillance methods. In Washington, AIDS lobbyists have requested the President to issue an executive order for the public release of documentation on known incidences of infection in the United States. Haseltine advocates widespread testing, stating, "Even AIDS researchers lose track of the scope of this disease," due to unreported and untracked cases of infection.

Haseltine's frank remarks countermanded the recently published analysis of the National Research Council, "The Social Impact of AIDS." The Council report stated that the epidemic would be self-contained within certain narrow geographic and cultural parameters, with the larger population sharing little risk compared to groups in which the disease is endemic. Regarding the development of a vaccine or a cure, Haseltine cautioned, "People are lulled by medicine. They think most things are possible. That isn't true. We have only a fraction of the knowledge that is necessary to cope with AIDS." He further stated that it is impossible to determine realistically if or when a vaccine or cure will be found. Yet Haseltine believes that the scientific community has mounted a successful mobilization against AIDS, noting that professional literature abounds with reports from all fields of science. One in twenty articles in the journals *Nature* and *Science* deal with AIDS, and one-third of the articles in virology journals address HIV, even though it is only one of hundreds of human infectious viruses.

Haseltine concluded his address with a warning: "Restoring the health of HIV positive individuals without eliminating their ability to infect others would be a disaster for society, because it would almost certainly increase the spread of HIV. We're in it for the rest of our lives, the rest of our children's lives."

Censorship by Intimidation:
Point/Counterpoint with Martin Delaney
(3/25/93)

In March 1993, Martin Delaney, Founding Director of Project Inform, wrote to The Sentinel, *complaining about my coverage of AIDS medical developments. The letter is reproduced below in its entirety, followed by my rebuttal.*

Letter from Martin Delaney

Dr. Donald Abrams does not deserve to be the subject of this week's tongue lashing by Charles Caulfield. Whatever his views on any particular subject, Dr. Abrams is a man of integrity who has been a tireless fighter and a pioneer in this epidemic. Ditto for Marcus Conant, Larry Waites, and all the others Caulfield has recently chosen to vomit on. He/they shouldn't have to take crap from Caulfield, whose attacks have become as predictable as they are unfounded and scientifically misleading. Sooner or later, someone must ask what give him the right, the credibility, or the imperative to use *The Sentinel* as a personal whipping post against everyone who disagrees with his eccentric views on AIDS. Caulfield has been the source of more misleading and out-of-context information on AIDS than any community columnist in memory. He conveniently lifts words and phrases out of legitimate scientific articles, twisting them to support his own views, much like the Bible-quoting fundamentalists who can find the answer to anything in their little black book, just as long as they're allowed to cut and paste any way they choose, Many of the scientific sources Caulfield quotes are horrified that their work is being misappropriated and distorted to support his views.

It is not Donald Abrams, Marcus Conant, and Larry Waites who are endangering this community, but irresponsible writers who disguise their personal anger and emotion about AIDS as "scientific" information and mislead people who don't have time to read and check the references they quote and so routinely distort. AIDS cannot be reduced to matter of dogmatic faith about individual theories or treatments. It is a complex and constantly moving target as the information base grows and evolves, not a soap opera to be used for selling newspapers. Over the years, I've noted two characteristics which dramatically separate the quacks from people who are sincerely looking for answers amidst the uncertainties of AIDS: 1. the quack is angrily, emotionally, and dogmatically "stuck" on the treatment or theory of his own choice, bending every little bit of data to support a pre-drawn conclusion, and 2. the quack spends a disproportionate amount of energy damning the beliefs of others who fail to support his brand of medical religion. If Caulfield can't get through even a few consecutive columns without engaging in "slash and burn," perhaps he should see if this shoe fits.

There are many ways to make constructive contributions in this epidemic. Medical Jihad is not one of them.

Caulfield's Rebuttal

Dr. Abrams, Dr. Conant, and Dr. Waites did indeed deserve the criticism and questions they have received in recent months in my column. It was accurate and fair to report that Dr. Abrams prescribes AZT to his patients, yet in *BETA* and the most current *AmFAR Directory*, denies that it prolongs survival or increases quality of life.[31] I recently spoke with Alice Trinkle, Media Liaison for San Francisco General Hospital's AIDS Services Division, who stated, "Well, Donald doesn't think that they're good drugs, but that people should take them since there's nothing else."[32] Dr. Conant receives God only knows how much money from Burroughs Wellcome and other groups that want clinical trials on potential therapies. He's told his patients to expose themselves to UV radiation which is dangerous for those with HIV infection. Dr. Waites did *not* read the literature on UV light and supported a position on exposure to sunlight that was both wrong and dangerous.

It is sad and disgusting that Delaney's primary concern is saving the reputations of his friends in the medical community, rather than saving the lives of people dying of AIDS. It is widely rumored that the esteemed Martin Delaney is now working hand-in-hand with the FDA's

David Kessler to close down the buyers' clubs and other alternative source of treatments for those who have forsaken conventional treatments, such as those prescribed by the esteemed doctors he mentions in his childish and irrational diatribe. In recent months, Kessler has been active in efforts to exclude vitamins and nutritional supplements from the status of over-the-counter medicines, requiring prescriptions for vitamin C and other nutrients, thereby driving up prices and limiting their use.

Curiously, Delaney comments negatively on my references to published AIDS research. Yet, he conveniently fails to mention that all of my references are listed and documented so others can check them. Any article published in a scientific journal cannot be taken out of context, for any statement in it is a valid reference. Submissions of manuscripts to scientific journals are returned to the author for rewrite if they are perceived by scientific peers and editors to contain statements which could be ambiguous, misleading, or taken out of context.

Abrams, who Delaney characterized as the victim of my "tongue lashing," is treated much less kindly by Delaney himself in *Acceptable Risks*, a comical biography of Delaney and his associate Jim Corti. According to author Jonathan Kwitny, Delaney described Abrams as representative of all that was elitist and wrong about the American medical research establishment, and viewed him as a power grabber, capable of tossing a "paltry bone" in the form of the Community Consortium, to patients angry over lack of treatments.[33] Yet, now he comes to Abrams' defense. When I recently offered to interview Dr. Abrams to clear up any misinterpretations that may have occurred, he refused.

Life saving drugs and treatments do exist and are now available through the treatment underground. There is hard clinical data to support their effectiveness. But Project Inform chooses not to inform the HIV-positive community about these drugs, and insists that standard antiviral therapy is the best way to go. Yet, under Delaney's direction, Project Inform funded a successful study on DNCB conducted at California Pacific Medical Center, which resulted in striking efficacy data using cutting-edge RT-PCR and CD8 subset technologies. But, since DNCB can not be patented and would return no profits or contributions to Project Inform, the study was disavowed by Delaney as "boosterism." In so doing, he cruelly misled thousands of individuals who have blindly trusted him. For the past several years, Martin Delaney has been talking down promising inexpensive therapy options and talking up potential treatments that will result in maximum profits for drug companies, royalties for his scientific friends, and contributions to Project Inform. It is now astoundingly clear that people with HIV are not the foremost priority in Delaney's advocacy of certain treatments.

I have made the focus of "HIV News" to provide information on alternative therapies—affordable and nontoxic methods of maintaining health for thousands of people in San Francisco. I have not confined the focus of this column to any particular treatment or theory, and all the methods I have discussed have been supported by current scientific research. Despite this, Delaney accuses me of being a "quack." In reviewing *The Sentinel's* "HIV News" section over the last several months, I have largely focused on treatment options, both conventional and alternative. This has included in-depth coverage of multiple options, such as Rifabutin, Bitter Melon, antioxidant nutrients, vitamins and minerals, DNCB, Acemannan, Chinese Medicine, alternative treatments for CMV retinitis, vitamin C, and certain veterinary drugs. I have also consistently advocated a holistic approach integrating body, mind, and spirit.

In contrast, Delaney's fanatical certainty that Compound Q would work, resulting in endangering lives in an underground treatment study conducted without benefit of toxicity data, would appear to be more like the behavior of a quack.

Thousands of people in San Francisco are satisfied with the alternative therapies they use, and I am committed to using this forum to continue to inform the community on the background and availability of these treatments. My sole purpose is to help people stay alive. Survival, Mr. Delaney, remember that idea? What a concept, eh?

Other local journalists critical of Delaney have also been the recipients of his legendary tirades. Lisa Krieger, staff medical writer for the *San Francisco Examiner,* once criticized Delaney in an article and received a letter to her editor discrediting her and slamming the paper for giving him negative press coverage. *Bay Area Reporter* columnist

Michael Botkin reported that his editor received an abusive and blistering phone call from Delaney after he satirized his financial dealings. Delaney's attempted censorship by intimidation and name-calling, received by three local HIV news writers, reveals an intolerable pattern. I will continue to inform my readers of cutting-edge developments in AIDS research and about underground access to treatment options they won't likely hear about from their doctors. The gay press must not allow itself to be coerced into avoiding sensitive and painful issues.

In his book *Rethinking AIDS,* Robert Root-Bernstein states, "assurance in science comes only through elaborating of as many possible explanations can be imagined . . . that process has not been employed in AIDS research. The door on alternative therapies was closed before anyone had a chance to see how many rooms there were, let alone explore their treasures. We must research them now."[34] This view is shared by the majority of PWAs who have found a way to recover their health. The establishment physicians know about this treasure trove, yet most don't partake of it. Some brave doctors who do refute standard therapy, claiming to see longer-term survival in their patients who do not use antiretrovirals. Thousands of PWAs in San Francisco, including myself, have found ways to recover health and live against the odds using various nontoxic treatments. This information is of paramount importance to people living with HIV. Dr. Root-Bernstein reinforces this view by stating, "I would not be surprised if the most important innovators in AIDS research and treatment turn out to be peripheral members of the research and treatment communities."[35]

Silence equals death, Martin Delaney. Your attempts to dictate what is "fair game" in media reporting will fail, and the dialogue about treatment options will continue. Root-Bernstein writes that in observing people who have survived full-blown AIDS for a decade or more, he noted that few had been treated according to the regimen touted by the mainstream. "Rather than taking AZT or ddI, many of these men have taken as few pharmacological agents as possible, and turned to herbal medicine and holistic health cures." And, he suggests, we would be wise to note that throughout the history of scientific investigation, "the greatest medical breakthroughs . . . were all met, initially, with total skepticism from the medical community."[36]

AIDS Research: A New Low
(3/25/93)
Billi Goldberg

Since the dawning of the Age of AIDS, theories have come and gone, but one premise remains constant: the media exposure of new theories is inversely proportional to their rationality and importance. The *New York Times* and its erstwhile medical reporter, Gina Kolata (doctor and stenographer for the AIDS establishment), have outdone their previous efforts.

In her recent article, "New Theory Suggests Cell Regulator May Hold the Key to Fighting AIDS," Kolata reaches the lowest depths of medical reporting.[37] Kolata relates how Leonard M. Adleman (University of Southern California) and David Wofsy (University of California at San Francisco) are proposing that AIDS is a result of an imbalance in the ratio of CD4 cells to CD8 cells. As Ms. Kolata's rendition of the facts is so garbled, I will instead refer directly to her source, an article by L. M. Adleman and D. Wofsy in the *Journal of AIDS*.[38]

Reseachers Adleman and Wofsy state, "Our hypothesis concerning T-cell homeostasis is as follows: In all cases of T-cell loss, whether selective or not, both CD4+ T-cells and CD8+ T-cells will be produced until the absolute T-cell count returns to normal, even if this produces or exacerbates abnormalities in the absolute CD4+ T-cell count and absolute CD8+ T-cell count. Put less formally, our hypothesis asserts that the T-cell homeostatic mechanism recognizes total T-cells and is 'blind' to the distinction between CD4+ T-cells and CD8+ T-cells. T-cell regeneration is initiated by a low T-cell count and ceases when the T-cell count returns to normal, irrespective of the CD4+ T-cell count and CD8+ T-cell count."

Frighteningly, this theory focuses on a supposed natural homeostatic process, applies it to HIV/AIDS, and then suggests that "depletion of all CD8+ T-cells is not necessary. It is only necessary to deplete enough cells so that eventually the CD4+ T-cell count returns to normal." Now the scientists propose to use their tweezers and remove

31

just enough cells so that the CD4 cells return to the normal range. The specific immunological purpose of all these CD4 and CD8 cells are of no importance; all that matters is to get the counts back to normal, or at least to a normal ratio of 1.5 : 1.

All this hypothesis means that Adleman and Wofsy have no idea why there is a selective depletion of CD4+ cells in HIV/AIDS. They ignore the fact that only 2 percent of the lymphocytes are in the blood, and base their theory only on peripheral blood counts. Because outdated and artifactual research has shown only a few CD4+ cells are infected, they disregard immunological research explaining CD4+ depletion. The fact that a large percentage of cells in the lymphoid tissues, for example, macrophages, dendritic cells, and follicular dendritic cells, are infected with HIV is cast aside.[39] The authors conveniently ignore that destruction of HIV-infected CD4 cells is a normal immune response. Furthermore, antibody and autoimmune (autoantibody) reactions against CD4 cells, along with clonal deletion and anergy, are deemed inconsequential in their "grand hypothesis."

These innovative AIDS researchers have laid aside all the research by dedicated and knowledgeable immunologists over the years, and have started the AIDS ballgame over from scratch. They noticed that in AIDS, CD4s go up and down and CD8s go up and down, and they are replaced in unequal numbers by the dysfunctional immune system. Their simplistic answer is to maintain the "normal" CD4 : CD8 ratio at 1.5 : 1. If there are too few CD4 cells, then raise the CD4 numbers; if there are too many CD8 cells, then lower that number. (Is it possible the authors consider three total CD4 cells to two total CD8 cells a normal ratio?)

In the lead editorial to this "blue-sky" article,[40] authors Stanley and Fauci state that "Adleman and Wofsy present data from a single mouse experiment that supports this theory," adding, "Such a novel therapeutic approach must be accompanied by several caveats, the first of which is to stress the fact that additional experimental evidence must first be accumulated to support the existence of this homeostatic mechanism." Finally, Stanley and Fauci state that "Depletion of these suppressive cells might theoretically accelerate viral replication and disease progression."

In science, simplicity is elegant, but to ignore past research is sheer ignorance. Adleman and Wofsy imprudently ignore the field of immunology and all that has been learned over the decades. The immune system is not a thermostat that can be turned on and off to regulate T-cell counts, but acts and reacts to infections and other abnormalities by increasing and decreasing antibodies, effector, and helper cells. In addition to these specific cellular responses, the immune system eliminates pathogens and abnormal cells and controls inflammation by phagocytosis, cytotoxicity, hypersensitivity, complement, and cytokines.

But we should not judge Adleman and Wofsy too harshly; after all, they just presented another meaningless theory to go along with the thousands of other meaningless theories printed in scientific journals during the last twelve years. The real blame for this situation should be reserved for medical stenographers like Gina Kolata, who publicize the trivial and ignore the few important articles that do emerge, such as Fauci's "The immunopathogenesis of human immunodeficiency virus infection" in the February 4, 1993 edition of the *New England Journal of Medicine*.

Time and time again, the media presents ridiculous theories that give false hope to thousands of people infected with HIV. Isn't it about time to stop proposing and publicizing theories and treatments that result in depression of the immune system, and start finding ways to boost the immune system to destroy HIV and the opportunistic infections that lead to the death of people with AIDS?

Concorde Study Topples the AZT Apple Cart
(4/8/93)

Early treatment with AZT is worthless and CD4 counts are meaningless as a sign of disease progression. These are the new findings from an interim analysis of the lengthiest and largest AZT clinical trial ever conducted, the so-called "Concorde" study conducted over three years by French and British researchers. The results were reported by the research team in a letter published in the April 3, 1993 edition of *The Lancet*, a British medical journal.[41]

AIDS activists and physicians were quick to respond to the controversial report which scientifically disproves the value of early intervention with antiretroviral drugs, the mainstay of HIV treatment in the United States. Paul Volberding, M.D., of San Francisco General Hospital, who pioneered the practice of early antiviral therapy, conducted a one-year study of AZT use in nearly 1,300 asymptomatic seropositive subjects with fewer than 500 CD4s. The results of his study, ACTG019, were reported in the April 5, 1990 *New England Journal of Medicine.*[42] This study was a logical progression from Margaret Fischl's questionable AZT clinical trial, ACTG016, that resulted in the approval of AZT.[43] The Concorde trial, by contrast, lasted three years and involved almost 1,800 subjects. The *New England Journal of Medicine* reported that Volberding's study found that various doses of AZT, ranging from 500 to 1,500 mg. per day, delayed the onset of symptoms and elicited noteworthy increases in CD4s. He reportedly deemed the trial too short to determine survival data.

Volberding, whose influential study has affected the care of thousands of HIV-positive persons in the United States since 1990, stated in the April, 1990 issue of the *Bulletin of Experimental Treatments for AIDS* that "Therapy with AZT is recommended for both symptomatic and asymptomatic HIV-infected individuals whose CD4 counts are below 500 at a dose of 500 mg. per day." The Concorde team, on the other hand, states unequivocally that their trial results "do not encourage early use of zidovudine (AZT) in asymptomatic HIV infected individuals."[44]

The Concorde participants, all of whom were asymptomatic seropositives, were randomly divided into two separate cohorts, with one group receiving a daily dose of 1,000 mg. of AZT, while the other was given placebo. If participants in the placebo group developed symptoms or experienced lowered CD4 counts, they were allowed to enter the AZT group. Throughout the study's duration, the investigators were not able to observe any significant difference in the rapidity of the onset of symptoms or in length of survival between the two groups, even after several interim analyses.

The subjects who took AZT experienced a marginal CD4 count elevation of about thirty cells at three months and thereafter, but no other clinical benefit. This was the only difference observed between the two study populations, leading the Concorde researchers to a conclusion which may have more importance to general AIDS research than their AZT data. They discovered that CD4 increases seen in the AZT group appeared to be irrelevant in evaluating an antiviral drug's effectiveness, noting that it does not correlate with any clinical benefit. The premise that CD4s are artifactual and do not correlate accurately to disease progression or improvement has been a focal point in recent months in "HIV News." I have advocated a shift toward measurement of CD8 absolute numbers and activation as true prognostic tools.

In a recent article, the *San Francisco Chronicle* quoted Volberding predictably disputing the Concorde findings, citing questionable flaws in the study design.[45] "First of all," Volberding stated, "the patients who participated from 1988 through 1991 took nearly double the dose of AZT commonly used today." The relevance of this seemingly inane statement becomes questionable in light of the fact that in his asymptomatic trial, ACTG019, the dosage range used was 500 to 1,500 mg. per day. Volberding also criticized the study's use of AZT alone, since the standard regimen used today also includes ddI and ddC. However, what is in current use today is irrelevant. The point is that the widespread clinical trial that resulted in standard use of antiretroviral drugs in healthy HIV-positive individuals claimed results which were not reproducible in a larger, longer, and very similar study.

Dr. Volberding has not reported the CD8 counts of the trial participants. In two attempts, I failed to obtain them from Volberding, who probably has good reason to suppress them. The journal *AIDS* reported an Italian study showing that CD8 counts decrease with AZT usage in both 500 mg. and 1,000 mg. doses during a six-month period with patients who had median CD4 counts of 424.[46] At the end of six months, the 1,000 mg. dosage group had their CD8 counts drop 120 cells, while in the 500 mg. group, the drop was sixty cells. High numbers of cytotoxic T-lymphocytes are the key to survival in AIDS; any treatment that decreases their value will result in speedier disease progression and resultant increases in opportunistic infections.

The only beneficiaries of the widespread use of AZT have been the treatment advocates funded by Burroughs Wellcome and financially motivated scientists and doctors who have made money from the pharmaceutical corporate giant. Marcus Conant, promptly and predictably, appeared on local television news to enunciate the flaws of the Concorde study and to advise "early intervention" patients to remain calm and continue to take their antiviral drugs. Conant clarified his position recently in the *Bay Area Reporter,* stating, "Unfortunately, the Concorde study shows no survival benefit with the use of AZT at the end of three years. That's no revelation to people in San Francisco. That's why we've been combining treatment all along."[47]

Conant, along with Volberding, has served as a clinical investigator for numerous Burroughs Wellcome drug trials. He has recently elected to withhold thousands of dollars of advertising from *The Sentinel* due to recent articles in which I expressed criticism of his treatments and clinical trials. Conant was also angered by my unmitigated gall in asking Donald Abrams, a revered guest speaker at a Conant forum, about AZT's efficacy in delaying symptoms and prolonging life. Conant wields a hefty advertising and public relations budget through the generosity of Burroughs Wellcome, and has now decided to direct those advertising dollars away from any media forum critical of his views. This is a blatant attempt to dictate editorial policy through financial coercion as a hedge against further criticism.

As the medical establishment goes on the defensive, activist groups are seizing the opportunity to decry the imprudent and dangerous use of AZT. In March, 1993 at the United Nations Human Rights Commission in Geneva, the Los Angeles-based advocacy group Project AIDS, International presented evidence of conspiracy and dissemination of false evidence of AZT's effectiveness in encouragement of "early intervention" with a known toxic chemical.

Project AIDS, International seeks to contact individuals who have lost a loved one to AZT, or who themselves have suffered the effects of "early intervention" with AZT. Spokesperson Mark Alampi stated, "You need to know your rights. Ask yourself the following questions: Were you mislead by the U.S. studies or information that was given you through the FDA or CDC? Were you pressured into taking AZT (read 'early intervention') by your doctor or an AIDS organization? Do you have any literature recommending early intervention or the taking of AZT as soon as you get your positive test results and when your T-Cells are lower than 500? If you have answered yes to any or all of the above questions, you have a right to compensation for wrongful death, product liability, medical malpractice, pain and suffering, and mental distress."[48] Alampi added that physicians can be held individually liable for development of AZT-related problems, such as anemia, bone marrow and organ toxicity, and peripheral neuropathy, as well as other AZT-related side effects.

As *San Francisco Chronicle* writer Sabin Russell aptly put it, "early treatment with AZT seemed to have no effect at all."[49] Physicians are likely to soon be compelled by necessity (and threats of malpractice litigation) to embrace new diagnostic technologies in order to evaluate the condition of their patients and the effect of the drugs they prescribe.

The AZT Plot Thickens
(4/15/93)

The circumstances surrounding the release of the recent European Concorde AZT trial results,[50] as well as facts obtained through independent research by Los Angeles based Project AIDS, International, clearly infer a conspiracy by Burroughs Wellcome to push the sale of their drug AZT. With a frightening toxicology profile, AZT has proven useless in the treatment of AIDS.

Two days before Project AIDS, International's report to the United Nations Human Rights Commission concerning the toxicity of AZT, the statistician analyzing the data for the Concorde study was killed in what has been described as a "suspicious" automobile accident. Dr. Ian Weller, principal investigator of the study team, decided to release the data as rapidly as possible. Realizing the ramifications of their findings, they feared attempts to suppress the release of the data, and likely feared for their personal safety as well.

The *Bay Area Reporter* recently reported that Marcus Conant, M.D., who operates one of the worlds largest AIDS private practices and is a frequent investigator for Burroughs Wellcome drug trials, stated that the Concorde trial showed AZT was less toxic than previously thought.[51] I beg to differ with Conant's rationalization.

A 1991 Harvard study on the immunosuppressive properties of antiviral drugs showed that AZT, ganciclovir, and ribavirin inhibited the proliferation of lymphocytes and impaired other immune functions.[52] In a letter in the April, 1993 issue of the *Annals of Internal Medicine,* two researchers stated that AZT has been shown to inhibit proliferation of immune cells and to diminish their responsiveness, and that AZT's effects resembled those of corticosteroids and other immunosuppressive agents.[53] Reseachers Macleod and Hammer, whose paper, "Zidovudine [AZT]: Five Years Later," appeared in an earlier issue of the *Annals of Internal Medicine,*[54] essentially concur with these observations in a letter appearing in the same edition of the journal.[55] In addition, researchers at at the National Cancer Institute showed that AIDS patients with fifty or fewer CD4s on AZT therapy had a life expectancy of one year or less.[56]

Yet CD8 counts, which have been clearly linked to immune activation leading to improved health and longevity in AIDS patients, have not been reported in any AZT efficacy trial to date. Investigators have repeatedly ignored attempts by myself and others to obtain them. Since Concorde concluded that peripheral blood CD4 counts were worthless markers, the CD8 data from Volberding's earlier and recent AZT trials must be released now. There no longer remains any doubt about the correlation between high CD8 counts and the ability to fight infection, and thus the value of these laboratory measurements. If Volberding has prognostic data pertaining to the efficacy of a drug which is now clinically relevant to his earlier findings, he has a public responsibility to release this data. AZT use demonstrably results in declines in CD8s in a dose dependent manner.[57] It's no mystery why these Burroughs Wellcome investigators do not want this information made available.

Jeremy Selvey, CEO of Project AIDS, International, stated that the organization has also been attempting to obtain CD8 values from antiviral trials. Over the last three years, they have repeatedly requested this information from David Barry, President of Research for Burroughs Wellcome. During their last contact with Barry six months ago, they were told that all material pertaining to their inquiries were under review in the legal department. Project AIDS, International's attempts to obtain this information from Aleister Fromer, Chairman of the

Board of Burroughs Wellcome, were equally fruitless. The group is currently attempting to obtain the CD8 data from the Concorde trial.

Dr. Volberding will discuss "The Future of Antiviral Therapy" in a public forum sponsored by University of California at San Francisco AIDS Health Project this month. A few relevant questions he will no doubt face are, "Where are the CD8 counts from ACTG019?", "If they weren't measured, why not?", and, "If CD4s were found by Concorde to be inconsequential, at least in evaluating antiviral drug therapies, what measures do we now have to determine clinical course and drug efficacy?" These questions are central to the future of antiviral therapies.

Three excellent references for further information on the many controversies surrounding the use of AZT are *Good Intentions* by Bruce Nussbaum,[58] and two books by John Lauritsen, *Poison by Prescription: The AZT Story*[59] and *The AIDS War.*[60] To join the fight to recall AZT, contact Project AIDS, International, AIDS Fraud Investigation Team, 8033 Sunset Boulevard, #2640, Los Angeles CA 90046; (213) 857-0809.

Gallo and Volberding Reverse Position on CD4s as AIDS Markers (5/6/93)

Despite the irregular circumstances surrounding the reporting of the AZT Concorde Trial, one point was clearly made: regardless of the usefulness of AZT in early intervention, the value of CD4 counts in assessing drug efficacy was bluntly discounted. The implications of this discovery is of paramount importance to future drug trials. This new perspective on T-helper cells is gaining increasing consensus among leading AIDS researchers, including Robert Gallo and more recently, San Francisco General Hospital's Paul Volberding. Both men have conceded that due to the apparent flaws in the current practice which rely upon blood measurements, more accurate indicators of immune status must be developed and employed in AIDS treatment,

Despite the clinical implications of such a discovery, The ever conservative John S. James states in the current edition of *AIDS Treat-*

ment News that "the conclusion that Concorde shows that T-helper count does not work as a marker for testing new antiviral drugs is, as we believe, open to serious challenge."[61] I for one, am anxious to discover exactly what *is* this challenge. In the same week in which *AIDS Treatment News* published James' statement, Dr. Volberding admitted a disparity between CD4 increases and clinical improvement in patients taking AZT in an article in the *Annals of Internal Medicine*.[62]

Marcus Conant, M.D., a frequent investigator for Burroughs Wellcome trials, stated in a recent interview that the abandonment of CD4s as surrogate markers would require us to return to using death as an endpoint in placebo-controlled studies.[63] This myopic inability of physicians to see what is right in front of their faces has impeded any real progress in extending AIDS survival time, despite ten years of research. While Conant frequently pays lip service to the newer diagnostic technologies, he never publicly advocates their adoption as standard clinical practice. Conant occasionally mentions polymerase technology in his public forums, yet there is still no widespread implementation of this technology, which can determine the impact of drug therapies on the body's viral burden after only a very brief time. Why is this technology not being employed? If standard blood measurements are being called into serious question, it is incumbent on physicians to use other types of available and highly accurate diagnostic tools to interpret disease progression or improvement.

Physicians widely refuse to embrace other critical measurements, such as evaluation of lymphocyte subpopulations other than CD4s, and measurements of activation of natural killers cells and cytotoxic T-lymphocytes. These laboratory parameters are seldom looked at, despite the fact that the technology to do so is currently available in our own San Francisco General Hospital at a modest cost. It seems odd that Dr. Conant, while conducting a clinical trial of CD8 cell expansion therapy, remains unable or unwilling to see the diagnostic value of measurements of CD8 cells and their activation markers such as HLA-DR, for all of his AIDS patients.

Those physicians who have begun evaluating their patients' progress using these newer markers have reported a decided advantage in determining whether or not a treatment strategy is working. An attractive feature of using CD8 counts and activation markers as well as PCR technology is that the patient's response to therapy can be assessed in a relatively brief period of time, thus allowing for rapid changes in the therapeutic protocol if it is not working.

I surmise that physicians' reluctance to let go of CD4 measurement is critically tied to the endless AZT, ddI, ddC, d4T, analogue therapeutic approach in which they have been indoctrinated. As CD4s have become the mainstay of interpreting patient response to chain terminating drugs, if physicians now recognize the invalid status of their clinical landmarks their therapeutic options may also be called into question.

Recently reported research indicates the possibility that these new diagnostic orientations would not support the use of the nucleosides. Much more likely is that they would demonstrate a more realistic perspective on the true efficacy of these drugs. When weighed against the profound immunosuppression researchers are currently attributing to the use of nucleosides, I begin to wonder whether physicians are afraid that these new laboratory techniques will demonstrate that their current focus of treatment is wrong. In light of what is now known about lymph node involvement in AIDS progression, is antiretroviral therapy a dead end? Peripheral blood measurements of T-cell populations and viral load are not representative of total body viral burden. This has been stated again and again in the medical literature, particularly by Robert Gallo, Anthony Fauci, and Cecil Fox.

When Volberding spoke recently at a University of California at San Francisco-sponsored public forum on "The Future of AZT," he neglected to mention his recent article. This despite the fact that a discussion of the role of CD4s as surrogate markers constituted a great deal of the question-and-answer period. It is difficult to comprehend why a physician would fail to mention in a public educational forum his own published observations relevant to the subject at hand.

In his *Annals* article, Volberding states that "CD4+ lymphocyte levels should not be abandoned as a surrogate marker, but rather that additional markers should be identified." He concludes by stating—and yes, he actually did write this—"We are not implying that these markers should not be used for predicting long-term efficacy based on short-term results, but are cautioning that such predictions may not be accurate." It's beginning to appear that researchers are now looking for a marker to prove that antiretroviral drugs work, after almost six years of their use in clinical practice. This is suspiciously reminescent of a cart-before-the-horse approach, unconscionable when human lives are at stake.

National Cancer Institute retrovirologist Robert Gallo was recently quoted in the local press as stating, "CD4 as a sole surrogate marker is dying."[64] Rather than reinvent the wheel, it's time to adopt the currently existing diagnostic and prognostic technology, and get on with the inevitable change in direction in treatment research needed to gain control of this disease and restore normal life span. The technology already exists; so do the treatments. Sooner or later, in light of mounting evidence for a needed refusal of treatment initiatives, physicians are going to have to admit they were on the wrong track. Researchers and clinicians must begin to look in other directions using the discoveries of current immunology, rather than rely on the limited knowledge available in the early years of the AIDS epidemic.

Volberding has recently responded to my requests for access to other markers recorded in the ACTG019 trial, and he has stated that he is attempting to obtain the CD8 counts from that trial. He also recently received a request from Project Inform for information relevant to the concept of switching to absolute CD8 counts as more accurate surrogate markers. In response to that request, Stephen Lagakos, Ph.D., Harvard School of Public Health and statitician for the ACTGO19 study, wrote, "There have been other studies of T-cells, and some of these have shown CD8 cells to be predictors of risk." He added, "The 'Surrogate Marker' studies that I and others have done show that CD4 is not a *complete* surrogate marker in the sense that it captures *everything* about a drug that might affect clinical progression."[65] Whether they like it or not, Project Inform and practitioners are having to face realities in AIDS diagnostics that they have long and adamantly opposed. What Martin Delaney of Project Inform has referred to publicly as my "eccentric views on AIDS" are turning out to be views that must now be embraced to help save lives.

It should be noted that graphs drawn from the results of the ACTG019 study included in Volberding's *Annals* article show a marked drop in white blood cell populations other than CD4s in the AZT subjects. This indicates that, although CD4 counts rose and stabilized under AZT therapy, other immunologically critical white blood cells, such as neutrophils and CD8 lymphocytes, declined immediately and continued to drop, reaching a low point at week sixteen in the group randomized to take AZT. No such across-the-board leukopenia was noted in the placebo cohort of the study. Consistently throughout the study, those taking placebo had 8 percent higher total white blood cell counts than the subjects receiving AZT therapy.

More research needs to be done retrospectively on this particular study due to doubts raised about its findings by other research teams, as well as the apparent decline in host-defensive cytotoxic T-cells which can be surmised a priori from Volberding's reported findings. This has been demonstrated in published research.[66] It should also be noted that this trial data exhibited the same consistent drop in total white blood cells in the AZT group for the first several months of therapy, although the study went further into the data and demonstrated a dose-dependent decline in CD8 numbers as specific cells diminished from AZT use. The role of cytotoxic T-cells is critical to almost all immune defensive strategies.

Concorde certainly does need extensive evaluation before any of its results can be deemed conclusive. But, at the same time, a good hard look at Volberding's study is also needed before we can steer our way out of the quagmire of current drug therapies. New methods of evaluating their usefulness must be found, to allow us to find satisfactory means to extend survival time and enhance the quality of life for PWAs.

DNCB Study Results Reported
(5/12/93)

A report on the effect of the topically applied photochemical dinitrochlorobenzene (DNCB) as a treatment for HIV appeared in a recent edition of the *Journal of the American Academy of Dermatology*.[67] The article reviews the findings of a recent pilot study using the skin-sensitizing agent as a therapy for HIV disease, and offers a retrospective analysis of regular DNCB use in ten long-term AIDS survivors diagnosed for four years or more.

DNCB has been used as an alternative treatment for HIV since 1986. Since then, discoveries in the field of immunology have further clarified its apparent mode of action. Much more is now known about the chemical's ability to modulate the immune system then has been previously reported.

Dendritic cells in the tissue have recently been identified as the primary antigen-presenting cells of the body, and are now known to carry a significantly large portion of the body's viral burden of HIV and other disease-causing agents. Impairment of these cells' activity by the loss of delayed-type hypersensitivity is one of the earliest and most consistent symptoms of HIV infection after seroconversion. According to this recently published research, topical application of DNCB modulates the activity of epidermal Langerhans and dendritic cells, initiating a systemic delayed-type sensitivity reaction throughout the body.

A pilot study conducted as a joint venture by University of California at San Francisco faculty members and researchers at California Pacific Medical Center showed that weekly DNCB application was associated with consistent and significant increases in CD8 T-cell and CD56 natural killer cell populations.[68] Evidence of significant decrease in the bodily viral load of HIV was detected using Reverse Transcriptase Polymerase Chain Reaction (RT-PCR) analysis of serum samples from the study subjects. Clinical stabilization of all study participants was reported for the twenty-seven months of follow-up of those who remained compliant with the therapy.[69]

At the 1992 International Conference on AIDS in Amsterdam, local AIDS activist and registered nurse David Baker reported to the international press that DNCB is the most widely-used alternative treatment for HIV in the United States. Its low cost and easy access makes it available for widespread use. DNCB is one of the very few therapeutic agents that have been observed to have a direct impact on the generation and activation of cytotoxic T-cells, a goal of cellular immunology. CD8 clonal expansion trials are underway at several sites, reportedly showing promising results in some patients suffering from Kaposi's Sarcoma. DNCB appears to achieve this same goal without the need for invasive procedures and unnecessary expense. It has been used as an antiviral in human and animal medicine for years,[70] with demonstrated activity against some human cancers.[71] Its unique mode of action is unlike any other currently available mainstream or alternative treatment. It is a potent biological response modifier activating only the cell-mediated immune response, downregulating antibody production.

Dendritic cells, the premier antigen-presenting cells in the body,[72] appear to be jarred out of their inactive or anergic state by weekly application of DNCB, initiating intracellular destruction of infected cells by cytotoxic T-cells (CTL) and natural killer (NK) cells. By initiating a systemic delayed-type hypersensitivity, DNCB activates only the cell-mediated (Th1) immune response. National Cancer Institute Researchers Gene Shearer and Mario Clerici have shown that downregulation of the humoral, or antibody-producing (Th2), arm of the immune system is crucial to the development of any effective immune strategy against HIV.[73] By initiating a Th1 response, DNCB also causes the activation of macrophages. These multipurpose white blood and tissue cells can effectuate the destruction of cells infected by viruses and other pathogens. It has also been shown in two studies that DNCB activation of Th1 shuts down Th2.[74]

Next to dendritic cells, primed macrophages are known to be the most effective antigen-presenting cells in the body, as well as producing messenger molecules that signal lymphocyte production of Interferon-gamma (IFN-γ), a chemical messenger utilized in all cell-mediated immune responses. According to researchers, this activation results in a sequence of events that give evidence of profound, effective immune modulation. DNCB's ability to downregulate antibody production is a crucial element of the suppression of the Th2 response, noted by reseachers Clerici, Shearer, and Jonas Salk as an essential component of any successful defense against AIDS. This has proved a difficult goal to achieve in human medicine. If antibodies could protect individuals from HIV, their own antibodies, after seroconversion, would give at least some protection against the disease. This is not the case, however, and the suppression of Th2 (B-cell activation, and antibody production) is necessary to achieve a pure Th1 phenomenon in humans.

All attempts to test DNCB in a large-scale, significant clinical study have been halted by market factors. Since DNCB it is not patentable, there is no financial incentive and no industry support for formal investigation of its potential. This promising agent, which in small studies has appeared to arrest the progression of HIV disease in all subjects, is widely used in the treatment underground and has reportedly effected improvements in health in thousands of compliant users.

Although DNCB is still largely considered a "fringe" treatment by many mainstream practitioners, it certainly merits further investigation into its apparent ability to slow or eliminate decline in AIDS. Its negligible cost, easy accessibility, and lack of toxicity make DNCB a treatment worth serious consideration by anyone living with HIV. Recent research at the NIH has shown that there is no latency period in HIV infection, as was previously thought. Since the virus is continually replicating in the lymph nodes, initiation of treatment with DNCB is recommended by researchers as early as possible after seroconversion.

DNCB appears to offer a therapy that achieves the goal of generating and activating cytotoxic T-lymphocytes at a price relevant to the financial realities faced by many people with AIDS. Moreover, as this treatment strategy gains increasing acceptance as a necessary approach to controlling HIV infection, it has profound implications for the global impact of AIDS, a morally necessary consideration for any legitimate HIV/AIDS treatment. *For more information on DNCB, see Resource Guide, p. 154.*

AIDS and Antibiotics Part 1: Drug Resistance and Immunosuppression (6/2/93)

Scientific journals and the news media are filled these days with reports of diseases considered easily treatable with antibiotics that are now developing resistance to the drugs that once controlled them. The most publicized examples of this alarming phenomenon are multiple-drug resistant tuberculosis and AZT-resistant strains of HIV. Drug-resistant disease are well understood by modern medicine. Any first year medical student can explain that a resistant bacterial strain can transfer its resistance to other bacterial strains through resistance factors and transposons (transposable genetic elements). It is a public health imperative to prevent endemic levels of drug-resistant diseases through prudent prescription of antibiotics. A basic tenet of medical ethics requires that antibiotics never be prescribed before performing a "culture and sensitivity" test, a set of diagnostic techniques to determine the most effective antibiotic to be used and the briefest duration of treatment needed to control or cure the illness.

Unfortunately, this ethical requirement is commonly disregarded by prescribing physicians. *The Antibiotic Paradox: How Miracle Drugs are Destroying the Miracle,* a new book by Stuart Levy, M.D., a world-renowned expert on the use of antibiotics, describes clearly the inherent dangers of physicians' presumptive diagnoses and excessive use of antibiotics, antifungals, antiprotozoals, and antivirals.[75] The excessive use of antibiotics is emerging in the increasing drug resistances of formerly treatable diseases.

Levy's book points out a further complication to this threat. In most of the Western world, the majority of meat, poultry, and fish consumed comes from factory-farmed animals treated with antibiotics to keep them disease-free and saleable. The soil in a vast number of farms across the country is treated with antimicrobial chemicals to prevent bacterial damage to crops. Dairy cows are routinely fed antibiotics, resulting in milk and dairy products laden with antibiotic drugs in a chemically viable state. A large percent of vegetables are exposed to antibiotics and antifungals to prevent disease. Even without the medical use of antibiotic drugs, they appear to be a seemingly unavoidable and undeniably dangerous element in our diets. Drug-resistant microbes have entered the food chain and are transferring their resistance to the billions of naturally-occurring bacteria inhabiting our bodies.

Many of these "environmental" antibiotics have immunosuppressive properties that have contributed to the emergence of acquired and autoimmune disorders in the last two decades. This phenomenon has been widely understood by physicians since the late 1960s and early 1970s, due to the surprising emergence of drug-resistant strains of the microbe *Neisseria gonorrhoeae,* which causes gonorrhea. The sex industry that sprang up in Asia during the Vietnam War produced this phenomenon, and it continues to pose a public health problem to this day.

Many of the antimicrobial drugs used indiscriminately today as prophylaxis for HIV/AIDS opportunistic infections were originally intended to be used only for brief periods, for the treatment of specific disorders proven susceptible to a given drug through culture and sensitivity testing. The documented side effects of some of the more common antibiotics used in AIDS treatment have toxicology profiles that have never been subjected to any meaningful critical scrutiny. A close look at these drugs is long overdue.

Sales of such prophylactic drugs represent billions of dollars in commerce for the prescribing physicians, drug companies, and pharmacies. Is it any wonder that they have never been investigated? The amount spent on prophylactic drugs far outweighs that spent on nucleoside analogue drugs. While some research has been done into investigating the immunosuppressive properties of these drugs, many of them are used in new, untried combinations, under the common practice of polydrug prophylaxis for opportunistic infections.

Speaking out about this certainly isn't going to win me any new friends in the medical treatment community, but the issue is much too important to be obscured by politics or personalities. This information is so compelling (and the situation is so obviously influenced by profit motives) that the facts must be presented. I will let readers draw their own conclusions.

Fifteen years ago, a paper entitled "The effect of antibiotics on cell-mediated immunity" was published in the journal *Surgery*.[76] It reported that commonly used antibiotics had unambiguous side effects, including inhibition of cellular immunity, suppression of delayed-type hypersensitivity, decreases in lymphocyte populations, and interference with T-cell responsiveness.

Besides the immunosuppressive properties of antibiotics, antivirals' suppressive effects on the immune system have been identified and recognized by practicing physicians since the development of antiviral treatment strategies. These have been clearly identified and published in the medical literature. One example is a study reporting that AZT, ribavirin, and ganciclovir are potent inhibitors of lympocyte proliferation.[77] The result of this inhibition is immunosuppression.

Other research on human subjects has resulted in the following profile of drug-induced inhibition of T-cell production, showing the range of percentages represent the dose-dependent impairment of in vitro T-lymphocyte proliferation: [78]

AZT (Retrovir): 30 to 60 percent
Acyclovir (Zovirax): 34 to 61 percent
Amphotericin-B (Fungizone): 20 to 75 percent
Ceftazidime (Fortaz, Tazicef): 20 to 40 percent
Cephalexin (Ceporex): 30 to 95 percent
Chloramphenicol: 15 to 50 percent
Chloroquine (Aralen): 30 to 100 percent
Clindamycin (Cleocin): 15 to 70 percent
Clofazimine (Lamprene): 20 to 70 percent
Clotrimazole (Lotrimin, Mycelex): 20 to 100 percent
Co-trimoxazole (Bactrim/Septra): 26 to 95 percent
Doxycycline (Doryx): 36 to 100 percent
Erythromycin: 20 to 80 percent
Ketaconazole (Nizoral): 20 to 90 percent
Miconazole (Monistat): 15 to 99 percent
Ribavirin (Virazole): 35 to 90 percent
Rifampin (Rifadin): 25 to 63 percent percent
Rimantadine: 70 to 97 percent
Spiramycin: 40 to 80 percent
Testosterone: 12 to 98 percent
Tetracycline: 25 to 75 percent
Trimethoprim (Trimpex): 10 to 80 percent

This is only a partial listing of the drugs frequently used for lifetime duration in people with AIDS. Compounding the immunosuppression inherent in each of these drugs is the fact that they are commonly used in combinations of three or more. To this, add the drug toxicity resulting in bone marrow suppression and decreased production of lymphocytes and granulocytes. Regardless of the outcome of the debate currently raging on the value of CD4 T-lymphocytes in prognosis, 200 CD4s is generally considered the point at which polydrug prophylaxis, using treacherous, cellular immune-suppressing agents in an already immune-compromised subject, is prescribed. Such a treatment strategy fails to take into consideration that many individuals have extremely high absolute CD8 counts that provide protection against the intracellular pathogens predominant in AIDS. Western medicine's persistent orientation towards attempting to kill the offending organism rather than to stimulate the body's natural disease fighting mechanisms contributes negatively to this situation.

The data outlined above was obtained from limited research conducted on antibiotics and immunity. Clearly, this is an area of investigation which must be pursued further. Many concerned medical researchers have been held in contempt and scorned by their peers for the suggestion that "overmedication" of patients may be harmful. Often the patients so prescribed are generally those most susceptible to immune suppression. Overmedication of antibiotics could be a contributing factor to the decline and death of AIDS patients.

AIDS and Antibiotics Part 2:
Prophylaxis at What Cost?
(6/9/93)

Most of the drugs used widely in AIDS treatment to prevent the onset of opportunistic infections fall into the broad classification of "anti-infectives." These include antivirals, antibacterials, antifungals, and antiprotozoals. The use of most of these drugs, even in short term treatment of acute illness have been shown to have a negative impact on cell-mediated immune functions by decreasing lymphocyte populations and impairing T-cell function. Lifetime prophylaxis with unlikely combinations of drugs has not been evaluated for a possible synergism that may result in profound immunosuppression. Conceivably, these side effects could prove to be lethal to an already immune compromised individual.

The use of the tetracycline derivatives has long been associated with the frequent side effect of mucocutaneous candidiasis infections in healthy women. Now it is known that candidiasis, a common yeast infection, is one of the earliest and most definitive symptoms of immune suppression associated with HIV/AIDS. Here is an example of an AIDS-like phenomenon being elicited in a healthy human subject by the use of a seemingly innocuous medication. The result is that the patient requires treatment for the yeast infection with powerful systemic drugs that further impair cellular components of the immune system.

It has now been clearly established that cytotoxic T-lymphocytes and natural killer cells are the body's "heavy artillery" against infectious intracellular pathogens. Recent research has shown that absolute CD8 counts can safely and accurately be viewed as markers of risk for disease progression. The authors of one such study in the journal *Research in Immunology* stated that, despite CD4 counts, "Most patients were free from late opportunistic infections caused by disseminated cytomegalovirus and *M. avium-intracellulare* until CD8+ declined below 500."[79]

A striking and obvious conclusion is that the natural defenses against opportunistic infections are drastically impaired by the use of drugs intended to treat disease. As delineated in Part One of this essay, many of the prophylaxis drugs used frequently in AIDS patients with fewer than 200 CD4s cause profound decreases in T-lymphocyte proliferation. These drugs replace the body's own defenses by interfering indiscriminately with DNA and RNA synthesis in fast-replicating cells. The result of this interference is a depletion of defensive cytotoxic T-cells and natural killer cells. Artificial protection against pre-existing infections is used at the expense of the body's own defenses. What happens when resistance to these drugs develops? Prior to infection with HIV, such infections were controlled by the immune system.

Margaret Pouscher, M.D., of the Conant Medical Group and University of California's Mount Zion AIDS Clinic, has been characterized in the past by one of her associates as being "more conservative" than most AIDS physicians in her reluctance to routinely use common prophylactic drugs.[80] In a recent interview with Dr. Pouscher, she pointed to the use of fluconazole (Diflucan) as a prophylaxis for cryptococcal meningitis. "I don't use fluconazole routinely in patients with low T-cells [CD4 cells] to prophylax for Cryptococcus."[81]

Pouscher also stated, "At Mount Zion, where we see a very large caseload of AIDS patients, we may see perhaps two cases per year of cryptococcal disease. To prophylax thousands of patients against such a rare event is, I think, a mistake." Pouscher pointed out that fluconazole, an extremely useful drug in acute infections, should not be wasted by using it needlessly, thus running the risk of resistance to strains of dangerous fungal diseases which can no longer be treated. She adds, "We're seeing virulent strains of oral candidiasis in patients now who are currently taking the drug. Some of these infections will not even respond to treatment with Amphotericin." Amphotericin (commonly referred to by patients as "amphoterrible"), is notorious for its horrific side effects. Many doctors in San Francisco use fluconazole as a preventive against candidiasis—tantamount to using a cannon when a fly swatter would suffice.

In four-page full-color ads in prominent medical journals, Roerig, the makers of fluconazole, promotes its use as prophylaxis against cryptococcal and other fungal diseases. Millions of advertisement dollars are spent to convince the medical community that using this drug will prevent some possible future event. Not mentioned is the cost to the patient's immune system, as well as the actual financial burden. Due to large patient caseloads, most AIDS clinicians do not have time to regularly review the medical literature and keep abreast of rapidly shifting trends in diagnostics and treatment. Overworked physicians are acutely susceptible to the advertising campaigns generated by the drug companies and our friendly "village" pharmacies that purport to serve the community while raking in exorbitant profits. To put it mildly, retail prescription drugs are among the most highly marked-up merchandise in American commerce.

Besides the antifungal and antibacterial drugs and their drawbacks, antiprotozoal drugs, used to treat intestinal parasites, have been shown to significantly impair delayed-type hypersensitivity and cell-mediated immunity. Flagyl, often prescribed for chronic diarrhea presumed to be caused by intracellular parasites, actually inhibits the response which should control the offending organisms.[82]

Just prior to and during the earliest years of the AIDS epidemic, Flagyl was widely and indiscriminately prescribed in urban gay communities to treat endemic parasitic infections. Sexually-transmitted disease (STD) clinics in gay communities did a thriving business treating parasites, gonorrhea, syphilis, and herpes in the late 1970s and early 1980s. How much the repeated use of broad-spectrum anti-infectives contributed to the generalized immune suppression in our community, in which AIDS first flourished, may never be known.

But the process still continues, extending not only into the domain of prophylaxis against opportunistic disease, but into the antiviral regimes targeting primary HIV infection itself. The development of AZT resistance and AZT-caused immunosuppression in HIV is becoming clearly recognized as a consequence of widespread antiviral therapy. In 1987, researchers at the University of California San Diego Medical School reported that AZT and ddC (ddI and d4T are related drugs) did not inhibit HIV viral replication in macrophages which are known to be the largest reservoir and producer of HIV in the body.[83] At doses 100 times higher than those used therapeutically in human medicine, AZT and ddC, while supposedly inhibiting HIV replication in lymphocytes, did nothing to inhibit viral replication in macrophages. Monocytes and macrophages are believed to spread HIV throughout the body. This points to the frightening fact that in addition to antiretroviral drugs known lack of efficacy, they are inexorably contributing to the development of more virulent strains of the virus while further damaging the immune system.

Something is really rotten in the AIDS establishment. The pharmaceutical industry has one of the largest public relations budgets and, therefore, one of the largest and most effective lobbying forces in Washington, D.C., home of the FDA and the NIH. Can we really trust the industry most likely to profit from this disease to work in the favor of the people whose lives are most directly affected? Whenever it has been lives vs. money in the United States Scientific-Medical-Industrial Complex, which has triumphed, hands down, every time?

Enough Is Enough!
A Review of the Berlin Proceedings
(6/16/93)

Once again we have been subjected to the yearly ritual celebrating the scope and resources of the world's medical-industrial complex. For the ninth year in a row, this year's International Conference on

AIDS held last week in Berlin promised breakthroughs in the prevention and treatment of AIDS. And, as in years past, the conference ended with researchers and clinicians voicing collective dismay at their inability to grapple effectively with the AIDS pandemic, dashing hopes with rueful predictions of the future.

This year, the Conference consisted of over 15,000 "experts," largely physicians and scientific researchers touting their pet theories and putative treatments. In essence, it might be viewed as 15,000 closed minds assembled at a cost of millions of dollars—money better spent on the development of treatment strategies and prevention measures that actually work. Not surprisingly, this bacchanal of self-aggrandizement once again ended with a resounding thud that said: "this disease is more than we can manage." Is this conclusion one which requires the pomp and expense characteristic of these international symposia to discern? Hardly.

An honest admission of antiviral research failure, although disappointing, would be refreshingly honest. Such an admission might clear the ground for undertaking a new direction in treatment and prevention research. And much to the disdain and resistance of the old regime, a new paradigm in immunology is emerging.

Possibly the only good thing to come out of this year's Conference is the belated validation of a line of research pursued by isolated immunology scientists and followed closely in "HIV News." During the last twelve months, this forum has covered the role of cytotoxic T-lymphocytes in disease progression, the cross-inhibitory roles of the body's cellular and humoral immune cascades, and the need for a reversal in emphasis from antiviral strategies toward immune modulation.

The Sentinel and the "HIV News" column have allowed me to explore a line of reasoning light years ahead of anything else appearing in the popular press. Through this forum, an immensely educated readership has developed, the scope of whose understanding now far exceeds that of many AIDS physicians. This line of thinking has seldom been "politically correct," but the truth of it has been validated by a small yet critical cohort of researchers at the Berlin Conference. A shift in the way medicine views the immune system is imminent, foreshadowed by its emergence in the medical literature during the last year. But is a multimillion dollar international science fair really necessary to elucidate what has been clearly described in scientific literature, such as *Immunology Letters* and *Immunology Today*?

The following example which clearly illustrates the lack of progress in antiviral approaches might actually be funny, if it wasn't so eerie in its implications. John S. James, publisher of *AIDS Treatment News*, was recently quoted giving his impressions on protease inhibiting drugs: "This drug ought to be tried. If we had anything that was any good, it would be one thing. But we don't—and this may be better."[84] Could any statement better characterize the drift and lack of progress which has been the hallmark of mainstream AIDS treatment research? The Berlin Conference appears to have been no more than a celebration of collective medical egotism, leading to futility and death for millions, perhaps billions, worldwide.

Project Inform's Martin Delaney recently cautioned, "The biggest danger now is for us to come away from Berlin with a false sense of hopelessness."[85] There is, in fact, no falsity to the sense of hopelessness generated by one more year's dead-end research initiatives. The medical community remains intractably focused on flawed antiviral approaches, damning countless people to miserable deaths while protecting the investments of drug company shareholders. The sheer opportunity for pharmaceutical industry advertising at these widely-publicized events is, at best, pernicious.

With utter glee, drug companies finagle opportunities to provide funding for transportation and lodgings for so-called "treatment activists," in order to offset dissent and protest. This is just another example of the obscene low to which these "scientific" symposia have sunk. What is truly appalling is the extent to which drug companies have gained the acquiescence or even support of many who were previously their detractors. The situation is loathsome, and, literally, sickening.

Numerous physicians left the Berlin Conference early in disgust and anger. Many felt that participants were only interested in touting personal bailiwicks of "information" to convince other scientists of the virtue of their reasoning. Their focus was not whether their pet themes represented plausible options for stopping the spread of or alleviating the suffering caused by this killer disease. Physicians and researchers in the audience during scientific presentations, were observed using their cellular phones to call their brokers, eager to cash in on any unanticipated late-breaking developments. They were busy buying and selling stock, hoping to reap huge profits on any promising pharmaceuticals getting the collective nod from the research establishment.

Dr. James Curran, AIDS chief at the Federal Centers for Disease Control and Prevention, was reported to view this year's conference as excessive, at best. In light of its cost and dearth of benefits, he recommended that the international conferences be reduced in frequency to once every two years, with national conferences of AIDS agencies to be held in the United States on alternating years.

Let's take this a step further. Let's eliminate altogether the pretense of these international conferences that are merely glory-grabbing opportunities for scientists and doctors to hobnob with their fellow wizards. The medical community had better hope that Toto doesn't pull aside the curtain concealing their bogus operations to reveal the true status of its horrifying lack of progress.

The AIDS epidemic continues to insidiously spread, adding more and more deaths to the current toll of over 200,000 Americans, and countless others worldwide felled by this disease. It is increasingly evident that medicine, the healing science, is being superseded by the sciences of politics and economics. How many more must die to satisfy the prurient interests of capitalistic ventures that make a literal "killing" from this disease. How many people have gotten rich on the prospect of the PWAs' deaths? How many more will capitalize on the criminal neglect and suppression of information vital to any meaningful treatment strategies?

What is needed is a fundamental change in attitude on the part of scientists in general, and physicians in particular, in order for this disease to be contained and controlled. No evidence of such a change was apparent at the Berlin Conference, which made last year's abysmal conference in Amsterdam seem exciting by contrast. Despite repeated failures, the misguided (at best) and criminal (at worst) attempts to find the right combination of anti-retroviral drugs still dominates the treatment research landscape.

It's time to eliminate the International Conference on AIDS as a regularly scheduled event. If scientists cannot cooperate and collaborate across institutional lines in their own countries, how can we assume they will do so in the global arena? The scientific community's characteristic territoriality must be eliminated in our own back yard, before we can expect any concentrated global response to this disease. If a radical change does not occur, it is becoming self-evident that AIDS will inevitably result in the elimination of black Africa, black America, much of Asia, and over 50 percent of the gay men living in the United States, though few dare to publicly admit it.

If and when significant breakthroughs do occur, ad hoc symposia for review and discussion by the global scientific community are needed. Until then, this yearly raising and dashing of hopes becomes more and more tiresome. Let's let the Ninth International Conference on AIDS be the last of its kind, a monument to human greed and closed minds. The money, energy, and resources expended there could all be better used elsewhere.

Researchers State "We Were Wrong about AZT" (7/21/93)

Shocking flaws in antiretroviral strategies for treating HIV disease were revealed in a forum held on July 14, 1993 to update the Ninth International Conference on AIDS in Berlin. The forum was funded by Burroughs Wellcome, and included presentations by University of California at San Francisco Professors Jay Levy, M.D., Paul Volberding, M.D., Marcus Conant, M.D., and Constance Wofsy, M.D., as well as psychologist Tom Coates, Ph.D., and National AIDS Commissioner Randy Miller.

UCSF dermatologist Marcus Conant, M.D., a long-time advocate for the use of nucleoside analogue drugs, lamented the dismaying lack of evidence that these drugs prolong survival in AIDS—regardless of where their use is initiated in the progression of the disease. Conant stated, "It is now clear that AZT and other antiretroviral drugs do not work as far as extending survival time in AIDS." The Concorde study, along with other studies, including a European-Australian Collaborative Group trial[86]and the United States Veterans Administration Cooperative Study,[87] reported that this class of drugs has no benefit in extending life in PWAs, although they do seem to induce a transient retardation of AIDS symptoms for eighteen months or less. "You're left with deciding when you want your eighteen months of benefit— at the beginning or at the end," stated Conant. A recent study by AZT mavens Robert Yarchoan and Samuel Broder at the National Cancer Institute have found increased incidences of non-Hodgkin's lymphoma (NHL) in antiretroviral users.[88]

Dr. Paul Volberding, San Francisco General Hospital Chief of AIDS Services, was principal investigator in the ACTG 019 study on the use of AZT when CD4 T-cells fell below 500. Volberding stated, "We wish we could easily dismiss the results of the Concorde Trial based on flawed study design. But we can't—it was clearly a well-designed trial." When asked about the treatment potential of the use of immune modulators, Volberding noted that in his plenary address at the Berlin Conference, Dr. Anthony Fauci of the National Institute of Allergies and Infectious Diseases spoke of the need for this type of therapy and indicated that the contact sensitizing agent dinitrochlorobenzene (DNCB) is among the most promising of these agents under investigation.

Jay Levy, M.D., a University of California at San Francisco retrovirologist, spoke of the need to develop strategies for utilizing the body's CD8 T-lymphocytes in order to suppress viral replication in CD4 T-cells. This contradicts the present research trend throughout the country focusing on destruction of HIV-infected cells by the cytolytic, or cell destructive, activity of CD8s and natural killer cells. A discussion of natural killer (NK) cells, which have recently gained wide attention as being essential to decreasing the body's viral burden, was strangely absent at the forum. Levy failed to mention the now universally recognized fact that the largest percentage of the body's HIV infected cells is not CD4 cells, but antigen-presenting cells known as macrophages and dendritic cells. Suppression of viral replication in CD4 cells would do little to stop the spread of HIV throughout the body.

The presenters engaged in much discussion (albeit, rather uncomfortably) of the opposing immune cascades Th1 and Th2 as an important discovery presented at Berlin. Yet, none of the researchers

58

appeared to have a firm grasp of the mechanisms or implications of this line of research. Levy mistakenly spoke of Th1 and Th2 in reverse positions of their theorized functions. When asked about the process of impaired antigen presentation by macrophages and dendritic cells, Levy appeared to lack familiarity with this new model of AIDS pathogenesis, and became clearly annoyed at one questioner's persistence in pursuing this line of inquiry.

Dr. Levy continues to search in his lab, as he has for years, for an enigmatic, as-yet undiscovered cytokine (immune signaling protein) to support his theory of a cytokine that suppresses HIV replication. Researchers in cutting-edge immunology labs throughout the country have already identified Interferon-gamma as the cytokine responsible for the predominant Th1 state maintained by long-term survivors. What Levy does not seem to understand is that the predominant Th1 state will suppress HIV-replication in CD4 cells that are of a Th2 lineage. These cells are antibody-helper cells and require Th2-inducing cytokines (Interleukin-4, -5, -6, and -10) for activation and initiation of HIV-replication. We might conclude that Levy's misguided search for the mysterious cytokine is nothing more than a wild-goose chase for a nonexistent entity.

Interferon-gamma, as well as Interleukin-2, have been shown to have a direct causal relationship with the high level of CD8s now seen as the common denominator among long-term survivors. Levy conveniently failed to mention in his report that in order for any recovery from AIDS to occur, virus producing cells—lymphocytes, dendritic cells, and macrophages—must be destroyed by the cytotoxic activity of CD8s and the natural killer cells.

Dealing with psychosocial aspects of HIV disease, Dr. Tom Coates emphasized that the lack of effective treatment strategies underscores the need for risk reduction and behavior change in groups at risk. Condom advertisements on television and radio, as well as grassroots community education targeting the new demographic groups expected to be hit hardest by the disease, were identified as the clearest educational needs to curtail the ongoing devastation of AIDS in the years to come.

Held at the palatial Hilton Towers in downtown San Francisco, the symposium presented a strange and contradictory message. In a venue with the trappings of a wedding feast, the substance of the presentations were delivered with funereal gloom. The forum corresponded with the release of the most recent edition of *Treatment Issues*, the bulletin of New York's Gay Men's Health Crisis. This historically staunchly conservative publication stated that "the belief that AIDS could somehow be transformed into a 'chronic and manageable' condition through the right mix of nucleoside treatments was shattered in Berlin."[89]

In the same issue, Veterans Administration AIDS researcher John Hamilton reportedly stated that recent data on antiretroviral therapy did no more than "extend the scope of our ignorance,"[90] leading the highly-respected *Treatment Issues* to conclude that efficacy of nucleoside drugs in virtually all patient groups lack data that supports their use. The article also stated unequivocally that the studies leading to the licensing of AZT and other antivirals in the same class were designed to obtain regulatory approval, not to address the question of patient care.

Dr. Volberding was the most forthcoming among the forum speakers in his assessment of the dismal implications of the conclusions presented at Berlin. He stated that based on the evidence presented at Berlin, patients must now look within themselves and make an informed decision whether or not antiretroviral therapy is right for them. Both he and Dr. Conant must be commended, despite their many years advocating antiretroviral therapies, for finally facing the truth and recognizing the need for pursuing other avenues of research.

Dr. June Osborn, Dean of the School of Public Health at the University of Michigan and Chairperson of the National Commission on AIDS, placed the entire Berlin Conference in perspective in a recent edition of *The Advocate*. She stated, "As an old virologist, I always thought that the straightforward use of antiviral drugs as if they were penicillin would never work. There is no magic bullet that can be shot off to make it all be over. If the conference helped us all get over that illusion, we are all better off."[91]

Notes

Survival at Any Cost

1. O'Connor, T., Gonzalez-Nunez, A. 1987. *Living with AIDS: Reaching Out.* San Francisco: Corwin Publishers.

Acceptable Risks by Jonathan Kwitny

2. Kwitny, J. 1992. *Acceptable Risks.* New York: Poseidon Press.

New Controversy over HIV and Suntanning

3. Goldberg, B. 1992. Personal communication.

4. Wallace, B. M., Lasker, J. S. 1992. Awakenings ... UV light and HIV gene activation. *Science* 257:1211–1212.

5. Clerici, M., Shearer, M. 1993. UV light exposure and HIV replication [letter]. *Science* 258:1070–1071.

6. Conant, M. A. 1991. Future issues in AIDS. *Dermatologic Clinics* 9:597–601.

7. Duvic, M. 1991. Papulosquamous disorders associated with human immunodeficiency virus infection. *Dermatologic Clinics* 9:523–530.

8. James, J. S. 1992. ***** Warning: ultraviolet light may stimulate HIV. *AIDS Treatment News* 161:4.

Caulfield Responds to Physician's Rebuttal

9. Dobak, J., Liu, F. T. 1992. Sunscreens, UVA, and cutaneous malignancy: adding fuel to the fire. *International Journal of Dermatology* 31:544–548.

10. Roberts L. K., Lynch, D. H., Samlowski, W. E., Daynes, R. A. 1989. Ultraviolet radiation and modulation. In: Norris, D. A., ed. *Immune Mechanisms in Cutaneous Disease.* New York: Marcel Dekker, p. 170.

11. Simon, J. C., Tigelaar, R. E., Bergstresser, P. R., et al. 1991. Ultraviolet B radiation converts Langerhans cells from immunogenic to tolerogenic antigen-presenting cells. *Journal of Immunology* 146:485–491.

12. See in particular: Simon, J. C., Krutmann, J., Elmets, C. A., et al. 1992. Ultraviolet B-irradiated antigen- presenting cells display altered accessory signaling for T-cell activation. *Journal of Investigative Dermatology* 98(6S):66S–69S.

13. See James, J. S. 1992. ***** Warning: ultraviolet light may stimulate HIV. *AIDS Treatment News* 161:4.

14. Peterman, T. A., Byers, R. H. 1987. Seasonal variation in AIDS and opportunistic diseases. Washington, D.C.: *Proceedings of the Third International Conference on AIDS* WP 42 [abstract].

1992 and the Emergence of the New Activism

15. Abrams, D. I. 1992. On the matter of survival; Volberding, P. A. 1992. Is it possible to prove a survival benefit from early treatment? *Bulletin of Experimental Treatment for AIDS* November 1992:12–15.

16. McLeod, G. X. and Hammer, S. M. 1992. Zidovudine: five years later. *Annals of Internal Medicine* 117:487–501.

Cytotoxic T-Cells and Disease Progression in AIDS

17. McDaniel, H. R., Rosenberg, L. J., McAnally, B. H., et al. 1993. CD4 and CD8 lymphocyte levels in Acemannan (ACM)-treated HIV-1 infected long-term survivors. PO-B29–2179 [abstract]; and Stricker, R. B., Elswood, B. F., Goldberg, B., et al. 1993. Analysis of lymphocyte subsets in HIV-infected patients treated with topical dinitrochlorobenzene (DNCB). PO-B28–2140 [abstract]. Berlin: *Proceedings of the Ninth International Conference on AIDS.*

Present Focus of AIDS Research Is wrong

18. Kolata, G. 1993. Tests show infection by AIDS virus affects greater share of cells; a clue is found about how the immune system is damaged. *New York Times* 5 January, B6.

19. Embretson, J., Zupancic, M., Beneke, J., et al. 1993. Analysis of human immunodeficiency virus-infected tissues by amplification and in situ hybridization reveals latent and permissive infections at single-cell resolution. *Proceedings of the National Academy of Science USA* 90:357–61.

20. Koszinowski, U. H., Reddehase, M. J., Jonjic, S. 1991. The role of CD4 and CD8 T-cells in viral infections. *Current Opinion in Immunol-*

ogy 3:471–475.

21. Nixon, D. F. 1992. The cytotoxic T-cell response to HIV. Bird, A. G., ed. *Immunology of HIV Infection.* Hingham, ME: Kluwer Academic Publishers, p. 59.

22. Heagy, W., Crumpacker, C., Lopez, P. A., Finberg, R. W. 1991. Inhibition of immune functions by antiviral drugs. *Journal of Clinical Investigation* 87:1916–1924.

23. Rowland-Jones, S., McMichael, A. 1993. Cytotoxic T-lymphocytes in HIV infection. *Seminars in Virology* 4:83–94.

Fauci says HIV Latency Period "A Myth"

24. Pantaleo, G., Graziosi, C., Fauci, A. S. 1993. The immunopathogenesis of human immunodeficiency virus infection. *New England Journal of Medicine* 328:327–335.

Abrams Presents Contradictory Views on Antivirals

25. Abrams' presentation, held at the University of California at San Francisco on March 1, 1993, was the monthly forum of the Conant Foundation, underwritten by Burroughs Wellcome.

26. Abrams, D. I. 1993. Survival: the ultimate endpoint. *AmFAR AIDS/HIV Treatment Directory* 15 January, pp. 5–11.

27. Pantaleo, G., Graziosi, C., Fauci, A. S. 1993. The immunopathogenesis of human immunodeficiency virus infection. *New England Journal of Medicine* 328:327–335.

Zip Code Genocide

28. National Research Council. 1993. *The social impact of AIDS in the United States.* Washington, D.C.: National Academy Press.

29. Kolata, G. 1993. Report saying AIDS impact is small is causing dismay. *New York Times* 7 February, Section 1:19.

Prominent AIDS Researcher Makes Bleak Predictions

30. First published in Baum, R. 1993. Prominent AIDS researcher paints bleak outlook. *Chemical and Engineering News* 1 March:29–30.

Censorship by Intimidation

31. Abrams, D. I. 1993. *AmFAR AIDS/HIV Treatment Directory* 15 Jan-

uary, pp. 5–11.

32. Telephone conversation, March 23, 1993.

33. Kwitny, J. 1993. *Acceptable Risks.* New York: Poseidon Press, p. 204.

34. Root-Bernstein, R. 1993. *Rethinking AIDS.* New York: The Free Press, p. 372.

35. Root-Bernstein, R. Ibid., p. 363.

36. Root-Bernstein, R. Ibid., pp. 362–3.

AIDS Research: A New Low

37. Kolata, G. 1993. New theory suggests cell regulator may hold the key to fighting AIDS. *New York Times* 9 March, B6.

38. Adleman, L. M., Wofsy, D. 1993. T-cell homeostasis: implications in HIV infection. *Journal of AIDS* 6:144–152.

39. Embretson, J., Zupancic, M., Ribas, J. L., et al. 1993. Massive covert infection helper T-lymphocytes and macrophages by HIV during the incubation period of AIDS. *Nature* 362:359–362.

40. Stanley, S. K., Fauci, A. S. 1993. T-cell homeostasis in HIV infection: part of the solution, or part of the problem? *Journal of AIDS* 6:142–143.

Concorde Study Topples the AZT Cart

41. Aboulker, J. P., Swart, A. M. 1993. Preliminary analysis of the Concorde trial. Concorde Coordinating Committee [letter]. *The Lancet* 341:889–890.

42. Volberding, P. A., Lagakos, S. W., Koch, M. A., et al. 1990. Zidovudine in asymptomatic human immunodeficiency virus infection. *New England Journal of Medicine* 322:941–949.

43. Fischl, M. A., Richman, D. D., Grieco, M. H., et al. 1987. The efficacy of azidothymidine (AZT) in the treatment of patients with AIDS and AIDS-related complex. *New England Journal of Medicine* 317:185–191.

44. Press Release: Results from the Concorde Trial. 2 April 1993. London: Medical Research Council.

45. Russell., S. 1993. Study raises doubts about early use of AZT. *San Francisco Chronicle,* 2 April, A4.

46. Landonio, G., Cinque, P., Nosari, A., et al. 1993. Comparison of

two dose regimens of zidovudine in an open, randomized, multi-centre study for severe HIV-related thrombocytopenia. *AIDS* 7:209–212.

47. Conkin, D. 1993. Conant on Concorde: "So what?" *Bay Area Reporter,* 8 April, p. 17.

48. Alampi, M., Selvey, J. 1993. Litigation Query Based on Concorde Study. Los Angeles: Project AIDS, International 10 April.

49. Russell., S. Ibid.

The AZT Plot Thickens

50. Aboulker, J. P., Swart, A. M. 1993. Preliminary analysis of the Concorde trial. Concorde Coordinating Committee [letter]. *The Lancet* 341:889–890.

51. Conkin, D. 1993. Conant on Concorde: "So what?" *Bay Area Reporter,* 8 April, p. 17.

52. Heagy, W., Crumpacker, C., Lopez, P.A., Finberg, R. W. 1991. Inhibition of immune functions by antiviral drugs. *Journal of Clinical Investigation* 87:1916–1924.

53. Stricker R. B., Elswood, B. F. 1993. Immunosuppressive Effects of Zidovudine [letter]. *Annals of Internal Medicine* 118:571.

54. McLeod G. X., Hammer, S. M. 1992. Zidovudine: Five Years Later. *Annals of Internal Medicine* 117:487–501.

55. McLeod G. X., Hammer, S. M. 19923. In response [letter]. *Annals of Internal Medicine* 118:571–572.

56. Yarchoan, R., Venzon, D. J., Pluda, J. M., Lietzau, J., Wyvill, K. M., Tsiatis, A. A., Steinberg, S. M., Broder, S. 1991. CD4 count and the risk for death in patients infected with HIV receiving antiretroviral therapy. *Annals of Internal Medicine* 115:184–189.

57. Landonio, G., Cinque, P., Nosari, A., et al. 1993. Comparison of two dose regimens of zidovudine in an open, randomized, multi-centre study for severe HIV-related thrombocytopenia. *AIDS* 7:209–212.

58. Nussbaum, B. 1990. *Good Intentions.* New York: The Atlantic Monthly Press.

59. Lauritsen, J. 1990. *Poison By Prescription: The AZT Story.* New York: Asklepios.

60. Lauritsen, J. 1993. *The AIDS War.* New York: Asklepios.

Gallo and Volberding Reverse Position on CD4s as AIDS Markers

61.James, J. S. 1993. AZT, Early Intervention, and the Concorde Controversy. *AIDS Treatment News* 173:1–6.

62. Choi, S., Lagakos, S. W., Schooley, R. T., Volberding, P. A. 1993. CD4+ lymphocytes are an incomplete surrogate marker for clinical progression in persons with asymptomatic HIV infection taking zidovudine. *Annals of Internal Medicine* 118:674–680.

63. Kingston, T. 1993. The Concorde AZT Trial: Does It Fly? *San Francisco Bay Times* 22 April, p. 6.

64. Kingston, T. Ibid.

65. Personal communication via fax to Paul Volberding from Stephen Lagakos, 1992.

66. Landonio, G., Cinque, P., Nosari, A., et al. 1993. Comparison of two dose regimens of zidovudine in an open, randomized, multicentre study for severe HIV-related thrombocytopenia. *AIDS* 7:209–212.

DNCB Study Results Reported

67. Stricker, R. B., Elswood, B. F. 1993. Topical dinitrochlorobenzene in HIV disease. *Journal of the American Academy of Dermatology* 28:796–797.

68. Stricker, R. B., Zhu, Y. S., Elswood, B. F., et al. 1993. Pilot study of topical dinitrochlorobenzene (DNCB) in human immunodeficiency virus infection. *Immunology Letters* 36:1–6.

69. Stricker, R. B., Elswood, B. F., Goldberg, B. et al. 1993. Analysis of lymphocyte subsets in HIV-infected patients treated with topical dinitrochlorobenzene (DNCB). Berlin: *Proceedings of the Ninth International Conference on AIDS* PO-B28–2140 [abstract].

70. Lee. S., Cho, C. K., Kim, J. G., Chun, S. L. 1984. Therapeutic effect of dinitrochlorobenzene (DNCB) on verruca plana and verruca vulgaris. *International Journal of Dermatology,* 23:624–626.

71. See: Stjernsward J., Levin, A. 1973. Delayed hypersensitivity-induced regression of human neoplasms. *Cancer* 28:628–640; Levis, W. R., Kraemer, K. H., Klingler, W. G., et al. 1973. Topical immunotherapy of basal cell carcinomas with dinitrochlorobenzene. *Cancer Research* 33:3036–3042; and Truchetet, F., Heid, E., Friedel, J., et al.

1989. D.N.C.B. for malignant melanoma: significance in the treatment strategy. *Anticancer Research* 9:1531–1536.

72. Knight, S. C., Stagg, A., Hill, S., et al. 1992. Development and function of dendritic cells in health and disease. *Journal of Investigative Dermatology* 99:33S–38S.

73. Clerici, M., Shearer., G. 1993. A Th1→Th2 switch is a critical step in the etiology of HIV infection. *Immunology Today* 14:107–111.

74. See: Dearman, R. J., Kimber, I. 1991. Differential stimulation of immune function by respiratory and contact chemical allergens. *Immunology* 72:563–570; and Cumberbatch, M., Gould, S. J., Peters, W., et al. 1992. Langerhans cells, antigen presentation and the diversity of responses to chemical allergens. *Journal of Investigative Dermatology* 99:107S–108S.

AIDS and Antibiotics Part 1: Drug Resistance

75. Levy, S. B. 1992. *The Antibiotic Paradox: How Miracle Drugs Are Destroying the Miracle.* New York: Plenum Press.

76. Munster, A. M., Loadholdt, C. B., Leary, A. G., Barnes, M. A. 1977. The effect of antibiotics on cell-mediated immunity. *Surgery* 81:692–695.

77. Heagy, W., Crumpacker, C., Lopez, P. A., Finberg, R. W. 1991. Inhibition of immune functions by antiviral drugs. *Journal of Clinical Investigation* 87:1916–1924.

78. Descotes, J. 1988. *Immunotoxicology of Drugs and Chemicals,* Second Edition. Amsterdam: Elsevier.

AIDS and Antibiotics Part 2: Prophylaxis at What Cost?

79. Fiala, M., Kermani, V., Gornbein, J. 1992. Role of CD8+ in late opportunistic infections of patients with AIDS. *Research in Immunology* 143:903–907.

80. Marcus Conant, in presentation at a Community Forum sponsored by Burroughs Wellcome at the University of California, San Francisco, May 3, 1993.

81. Phone conversation with Margaret Pouscher, M.D., June 7, 1993.

82. Descotes, J. 1988. *Immunotoxicology of Drugs and Chemicals,* Second Edition. Amsterdam: Elsevier.

83. Richman, D. D., Kornbluth, R. S., Carson, D. A. 1987. Failure of

dideoxynucleosides to inhibit human immunodeficiency virus replication in cultured human macrophages. *Journal of Experimental Medicine* 166:1144–1149.

Enough is Enough! A Review of the Berlin Proceedings

84. Krieger, L. 1993. Promising drug curbs HIV growth. *San Francisco Examiner,* 11 June, A1.

85. Perlman, D. 1993. AIDS forum ends with focus on prevention. *San Francisco Chronicle,* 12 June, A1.

Researchers Say "We Were Wrong about AZT"

86. Cooper, D. A., Gatell, J. M., Kroon, S., et al. 1993. Zidovudine in person with asymptomatic HIV infection and CD4+ cell counts greater than 400 per cubic millimeter. *New England Journal of Medicine* 329:297–303.

87. Hamilton, J. D., Hartigan, P. M., Simberkoff, M. S., et al. 1992. A controlled trial of early versus late treatment with zidovudine in symptomatic human immunodeficiency virus infection. *New England Journal of Medicine* 326:437–443.

88. Pluda, J. M., Venzon, D. J., Tosato, G., Lietzau, J., Wyvill, K., Nelson, D. L., Jaffe, E. S., Karp, J. E., Broder, S., Yarchoan, R. 1993. Parameters affecting the development of non-Hodgkin's lymphoma in patients with severe human immunodeficiency virus infection receiving antiretroviral therapy. *Journal of Clinical Oncology* 11:1099–1107.

89. Link, D. 1993. The Collapse of Early Intervention at the Ninth International AIDS Conference. *Gay Men's Health Crisis Treatment Issues* Vol. 7, No. 6, p. 1.

90. Link, D. Ibid.

91. Bull., C. 1993. No news is bad news. *The Advocate* 13 July, p. 28.

Part Two

Alternative AIDS Treatments: Theories, Therapies, and Resources

Antioxidant Therapies for HIV
(7/16/92)

Oxygen is among the most abundant and vital elements in our environment. Along with sunlight and water, it is a fundamental staple of life on Earth. Traveling throughout the body carried by red corpuscles in the bloodstream, oxygen regenerates cells and tissues, promotes metabolism, and provides essential nutrition to the brain and other organs.

In its most common and useful form, oxygen occurs in the atmosphere as O_2 gas: two atoms of oxygen bound together in a stable molecular compound. In this form, oxygen, along with nitrogen, comprises a large part of the air we breathe. A single oxygen atom, O_1, is unstable, and over time produces damage to the cells of the body. Unbound to other single oxygen atoms, O_1 adheres to the surfaces of the body's internal membranes leading to cellular degeneration and increased susceptibility to illness. These renegade oxygen atoms, known as *free radicals* or *singlet oxygen*, have been shown to be damaging to the cellular component of the immune system.

A crude analogy for the harm free radicals can do to human tissue can be seen in the effect they have on metals. Iron exposed to singlet oxygen begins to deteriorate from the surface down, producing iron oxide, more commonly known as rust. Oxidative damage to the cells of the body is called lipid peroxidation, because it refers specifically to the damage done to the lipid, or fatty composition, of cell walls and membranes. There has been a great deal of research into the effect of free radicals on human metabolism. The concept was popularized some years ago by Dirk Pearson and Sandy Shaw in their best-selling book *Life Extension,* in which they argued that aging is largely a function of immune breakdown caused in part by the cumulative effects of peroxidation.[1]

Logically, people living with immune deficiencies ought to consider the possibility of taking measures to reduce the amount of damage done to their cells by oxygen free radicals. Many people do this by supplementing their diets with antioxidant nutrients and vitamins. This is a part of the approach to human illness known as Orthomolecular Medicine.

Oxygen free radicals are produced by several unavoidable factors in our environment. Toxins, highly processed foods, large amounts of saturated fats in our diets, and, significantly, stress can cause oxygen to degenerate from its stable and useful form. Antioxidant therapies seek to remedy deficiencies caused by these factors, decrease the damage done to the immune system and, speculatively, slow down the aging process.

Listed below are some items for consideration as adjuncts to ongoing medical care in managing HIV. However, shop around! There is enormous variance in prices for these items from distributor to distributor.

Superoxide Dismutase

Commonly referred to as S.O.D., this substance is one of the basic building blocks of the body's antioxidant response. It is usually extracted from wheat or barley sprouts. S.O.D. must be taken as *enterically coated* tablets, since it is not absorbed from the stomach but through the intestines.

Glutathione Peroxidase

This substance is a complement to superoxide, and they are often packaged in a combination tablet. In addition to its antioxidant properties, Glutathione Peroxidase has been shown in laboratory experiments to inhibit HIV replication. Several studies are currently underway to assess this potential in human subjects.

Beta Carotene

Also known as *provitamin A,* beta carotene is a nontoxic form of vitamin A that can be stored in the body. There has been much research establishing beta carotene as a strong anti-cancer agent. Known to inhibit several viruses in the test tube, it is theorized that beta carotene may help protect the epithelial cells in the linings of the lungs and those surrounding the major organs of the body.

Vitamin E and Selenium

These two minerals require each other to function optimally. They are essential to cell and tissue repair, as well as regeneration of damaged nerve tissue.

Germanium

This is a fossilized plant product used widely in Japan as a cancer preventative. A powerful antioxidant, it has been shown to increase the body's production of interferon, providing circumstantial evidence for immunomodulating properties. It is not absorbed well through the stomach, and is best utilized when taken sublingually (allowed to dissolve under the tongue).

Co-Enzyme Q-10

This is another nutrient used in Japan as an anti-cancer agent. It is vital to the body's healing and tissue repair functions, and increases the body's ability to utilize oxygen. It also appears to be useful in maintaining healthy heart tissue, decreasing gum disease, and strengthening the cell walls lining the blood vessels.

Vitamin C

This is probably the most widely used orthomolecular therapeutic agent, and also the most controversial. A powerful antioxidant, vitamin C is a staple in the intake of many long-term survivors of AIDS. It has a demonstrated antiviral effect but it is commonly believed by PWAs who use the therapy that *tissue saturation* level dosages must be consumed at regular intervals to utilize its antiviral properties. To achieve this, dosage is increased over several days until diarrhea occurs then decreased until symptoms abate, a process known as *bowel tolerance dosage.*

There are many more substances with greater or lesser degrees of antioxidant effects. It is not my intent to suggest changes in current treatment strategies, but rather to provide a basis for further research leading to informed choices. One superb reference on this and other relevant topics is *Living With AIDS: Reaching Out,*[2] by Tom O'Conner, a PWA who did a great deal of research into nutritional therapeutics. *Living With AIDS* is possibly the most thorough resource on HIV survival strategies available to date.

See Resource Guide, pp. 153–155, for information on this and other resources and supplies for treatment options, including both conventional and alternative therapies.

Acemannan
(7/23/92)

Carrington Laboratories in Dallas recently cleared several hurdles in their seven-year struggle to obtain regulatory approval for their anti-HIV drug, Acemannan, also known as Carrisyn. The USDA has granted Carrington a conditional license to market the drug for the treatment of Fibrosarcoma, a soft-tissue cancer in mammals. This disease is not unlike Kaposi's Sarcoma in humans, for which there is no available treatment.

This experimental treatment, under the name Acemannan Immunostimulant, is currently being distributed through Carrington Veterinary Medical Division in injectable form for the treatment of dogs and cats with Fibrosarcoma. The product license is conditional while efficacy studies are in progress. The company plans to begin clinical trials using Acemannan in the treatment of human cancers during the next twelve months.

Carrington has also obtained a license to market the drug as a vaccine adjuvant for the prevention of Marek's Disease, a viral disease in chickens that renders them unfit for human consumption. Marketed by Solvay Corporation under the name ACM-1, Acemannan will be used in combination with Solvay's MD-VAC vaccine. Solvay has indicated that this configuration provides earlier and more effective protection against Marek's Disease than MD-VAC alone.

Carrington scientists recently presented the results of a study testing Acemannan against Feline Immunodeficiency Virus (FIV), the cause of a disease like AIDS in cats.[3] The study findings were presented at the International Symposium on FIV at the University of California Davis. At the time of the presentation, Acemannan had produced significant increases in the infected cats' T-cell counts, as well as a decrease in the incidence of systemic bacterial infections. The clinical status of the FIV-infected cats improved with their prognosis for survival appearing to be substantially higher than those in the control group.

Acemannan is a complex carbohydrate extracted from the aloe vera plant. It has been shown to have a broad spectrum of action against viruses that infect warm blooded-animals and HIV in vitro.[4] Additionally, the drug has been shown to stimulate host immunity. Due to this property, Acemannan belongs to a new class of substances known as biological response modifiers. Unlike other complex carbohydrates that are digested and burned for energy, the Acemannan molecule is absorbed intact into the bloodstream where it accumulates in macrophages, multipurpose white blood cells vital to immune system function. After absorbing Acemannan, the macrophages have been shown to respond by increasing their production of vital immunologic protein substances, called cytokines. These include Interleukin-1 (T-cell stimulator factor) and tumor necrosis factor. These substances function to elicit the immune cascade of host defenses, including escalated production of natural killer cells vital to the body's ability to fight off so-called opportunistic infections. Acemannan has also showed the ability to enhance the allo-responsiveness of human lymphocytes in vitro.[5]

Acemannan has a long and convoluted history of research into its application against HIV, a process confounded by regulatory agency red tape as well as Carrington's lack of experience in the drug approval process. This is unfortunate, as pre-clinical animal studies as well as FDA-supervised Phase I dose tolerance studies in humans have demonstrated that Acemannan has virtually no overt toxicity. Carrington, a small biotechnology firm, has been no match for the pharmaceutical industry giants competing in the marketplace for approval of HIV treatments.

Between 1985 and 1988, Carrington conducted three uncontrolled FDA-sanctioned clinical pilot studies in human volunteers with AIDS and ARC. The results of these studies are on public record and are extremely encouraging. The initial investigation of Acemannan in AIDS treatment was conducted by H. Reg McDaniel, Director of Clinical Laboratories at Dallas/Ft. Worth Medical Center, in conjunction with the private practices of five Dallas physicians. Using Acemannan as the primary treatment for ARC and AIDS patients, the team observed significant results. Using a modified version of the Walter Reed Scale, designed by the Centers for Disease Control to define symptomatology, as well as T-cell subsets and the patients' subjective reports, they reported an overall 69 percent reduction in symptoms during the initial ninety days of therapy. T-cell counts increased significantly for the group, and circulating viral core protein (p24 antigen) levels were reduced or eliminated in the majority of subjects. This was accompanied by an average of two full Walter Reed Scale levels of improvement for the test groups.

Despite these encouraging results, Carrington has had little success in gaining attention for this drug in the United States. However, in countries with socialized medical systems, in which profit is not the determining factor for which drugs become available in the marketplace, Acemannan has received wider attention. In particular, the Canadian government has undertaken formal investigations of the drug for several indications. In 1990, the Canadian HIV Trials Network, a branch of Health and Welfare of Canada, underwrote a Phase II placebo-controlled efficacy study of Acemannan in human volunteers with symptomatic HIV infection. Earlier research by the Alabama-based Southern Research Institute, a contract drug screening lab used by the National Cancer Institute, found that in addition to stimulating the immune system, Acemannan acted synergistically with AZT, allowing the AZT dosages required to inhibit HIV replication to be reduced by 90 percent. Based on these findings, the Canadian government is currently testing Acemannan in combination with AZT in HIV-infected humans with low T-cell counts. It is theorized that this combination therapy will help maintain lymphocyte counts and reduce the toxicity associated with higher doses of antiretroviral drugs. In March 1992, the Canadian government's Health Protection Branch performed an interim analysis of the data compiled to date. Encouraged by the results, the agency recommended that the trial continue as outlined in the original study protocol.

In light of this information, we might ask why so little has been heard about this drug. It is likely that the relatively small size of Carrington Labs compared to its competitors has helped keep Aceman-nan out of the limelight, despite the fact that there is substantial pub-lished material on the drug in the medical literature. Acemannan's properties and mode of action have been documented in such jour-nals as the *International Journal of Immunopharmacology, The Jour-nal of Molecular Biotherapy,* and *Glycobiology.* But the AIDS activist press has been less attentive, despite the fact that this material has been repeatedly brought to the attention of both Project Inform and the publisher of *AIDS Treatment News* by myself and others since 1987. Unfortunately, awareness of Acemannan in the HIV treatment community remains minimal.

Carrington is able to make Acemannan available to the public in its raw form through a stabilization and preservative process. It is available in an aloe drink called the DeVeras Beverage, marketed under a private label by DeVeras, Inc. The known therapeutic equiv-alent is 1,000 mg. of Acemannan in twenty ounces of DeVeras Bever-age—the proposed daily therapeutic minimum dose to induce the desired effects. Since Carrington is still in the process of pursuing FDA approval for Acemannan, DeVeras makes no medical claims for its aloe beverage. *See Resource Guide, p. 153.*

Acemannan is only one of a new class of drugs called glycobio-logics emerging on the medical horizon. Most are extracts from plant gums and show a variety of systemic responses with little or no toxi-city. We are entering an age in which expensive toxic therapeutic agents are being made obsolete by more natural and affordable sub-stances. Carrington appears to have produced the most effective of these to date. It is unfortunate that the U. S. health care system and the pharmaceutical industry is so slow to explore this promising new area of study.

Delayed Hypersensitivity Therapy for HIV: DNCB
(7/30/92)

Since the earliest days of the AIDS epidemic, a number of promis-ing treatments have emerged on the medical horizon; most, on closer examination, have proved disappointing. Brought to the forefront by treatment activists, literally hundreds of new drugs have come and gone from public view, most having been little more than a "flash in the pan." A few, however, have shown remarkable longevity, and are as promising today as when they first appeared. Despite a lack of controlled research into their effectiveness, many people claim to owe their health, and even their lives, to the use of these remarkable therapies.

The skin sensitizing agent, Dinitrochlorobenzene (DNCB) is one such drug which has generated a continuously high level of interest in the treatment underground. DNCB has eluded the attention of the drug research establishment since it first came into widespread use over six years ago, despite some interesting and significant properties the chemical is known to posses.[6] And, unlike many treatment options, DNCB is also readily available and ridiculously inexpensive.

A library reference search on DNCB using MEDLINE revealed over 2,000 appearances in medical journals since 1966. The drug has a long history of pharmacological study and is known to be safe. Unfortunately, the primary characteristic of DNCB that makes it so attractive to those who could benefit from its use is, paradoxically, the same quality that makes the drug an unlikely subject for pharmaceutical research: namely, its low cost. Since DNCB costs less than two dollars per month to use, there is no profit motive to inspire research into this drug, despite its obvious potential in medicine. Even more inhibiting to corporate interest, DNCB cannot be patented.[7] Patenting procedures for drugs require that they be novel compounds. DNCB does not comply with this requirement, since so much is known about its composition and uses. So, even though DNCB may be a potentially lifesaving treatment for thousands of people living with HIV, with no promise of financial return on its development it is unlikely that it will come under formal investigation.

In spite of this, some physicians are continuing to look into DNCB and the patients who use it, notably Raphael B. Stricker, M.D., Associate Director of Immunotherapy at San Francisco's California Pacific Medical Center, and William L. Epstein, M.D., Professor and former Chairman of the Dermatology Department at the University of California at San Francisco. Both served as investigators in the clinical pilot study of DNCB's effectiveness. Their study, which was the subject of a scientific poster presentation at the Eighth International Conference on AIDS in Amsterdam, highlights the results of investigations surrounding DNCB treatment for HIV-positive individuals over an average period of seven months.[8] Favorable responses included significant reduction of reverse transcriptase levels using the Polymerase Chain Reaction Assay. Progression of symptoms was virtually halted for all subjects during the course of therapy, and no toxicity was noted except for the expected side effect of contact dermatitis at the site of topical application.

DNCB acts as an immune modulator through a unique mode of action. Its effects are limited to the cellular mediated component of the immune system. This approach is in keeping with the recently revised position of Dr. Jonas Salk, who stated in Amsterdam that he now advocates refocusing therapeutic approaches away from the antibody-producing activities of the immune system and redirecting them toward its cellular functions. This new rationale is further supported by recent developments in immunology, in which key immune cells on the surface of the skin and in the mucosal tissues have been shown to play a critical role in viral disease progression.

When applied directly to the skin at weekly intervals, DNCB activates the cellular memory, initiating a systemic migration of Langerhans/dendritic cells.[9] These immune cells, recently identified as key players in viral disease progression, act as sentinels for the immune response.[10] Traveling along these pathways from the skin and mucosal tissues to the lymphoid organs, they pick up HIV virions as "hitch-hikers." When these cells arrive at the lymph nodes, they present the viral surface proteins to CD4 T-lymphocytes, which in turn initiate destruction of infected cells and the viruses they carry. In this way, a significant amount of virus is removed from the body.

This process results in the generation of a new population of Langerhans/dendritic cells, and the cycle begins again. These cells cause a cyclical flushing out of significant amounts of the offending virus, and presumably any other intracellular infective pathogens. This "immune-bathing" of tissues from within may also reduce resident populations of all types of viruses, as well as bacteria, fungi, and protozoa.[11] To control enteric infections which are rampant in HIV/AIDS, immune responses must be initiated in the Peyer's patches

(PP), the lymph nodes of the small intestines.[12] This would explain the cessation of clinical decline for subjects in the pilot study.

This noticeable halt of the progression of illness symptoms was the most notable effect of DNCB in the study population. Additionally, long-time users of the drug report regressions of Kaposi's Sarcoma lesions and warts, elimination of thrush and other fungal infections, increases in laboratory measurements of CD8 T-lymphocytes, activation of natural killer cells, and a general resolution of subjective complaints.

While it is unlikely that formal trials of DNCB will be undertaken any time soon, many physicians and their patients are excited about the drug's promise. It is widely available in what have become known as "guerrilla clinics," and is currently in use by thousands of PWAs across the country. *See Resource Guide, p. 154.*

Natural Therapies for Candidiasis Infections
(8/27/92)

Candida Albicans, commonly known as thrush, is a yeast infection that grows in the mouth and throat causing localized pain and difficulty in swallowing. Undoubtedly the most frequently encountered infection among people with HIV, when Candida invades the esophagus it becomes an AIDS-defining illness, according to the Centers for Disease Control criteria.

Candida albicans is a natural resident of the body but it grows unchecked in the absence of an intact immune status, causing further damage to an already compromised immune system. While invading the system, candida produces rootlike structures called hyphae that penetrate the mucosa of the gastrointestinal tract, allowing toxins to enter the bloodstream from the stomach and intestines, and providing a route of entry for systemic invasion of the circulatory system. Candida is known to impair immune functioning by directly and negatively impacting the helper-suppressor ratio of T-lymphocytes.

While often effective, conventional therapies have serious drawbacks. Nizoral can cause serious liver toxicity; Diflucan is prohibitively expensive at nine dollars per tablet. Mycelex troches require the inconvenience of having to dose every three hours to get results. And Peridex and Nystatin get very mixed reviews from PWAs who frequently encounter this troublesome dilemma.

However, there are some natural remedies for the treatment and prevention of recurrent fungal infections. As with conventional medical treatments, these should also be used under the supervision of a licensed health-care practitioner.

Pau D'Arco

Also known as Taheebo and Ipi Roxo, Pau D'Arco is an extract from the bark of a South American tree, used for centuries by Incan cultures and the indigenous and local residents of its native region. It is known to have potent antifungal properties, and there is circumstantial evidence that Pau D'Arco has immunostimulatory and anti-tumor properties as well. It is very affordable and is available from most health food retailers.

Pau D'Arco is used in an infusion of the shredded bark, which is available in bulk or in tea bags. Argentinian Pau D'Arco is preferable to the Brazilian variety, as Brazil uses toxic pesticides. A strong tea of Pau D'Arco, taken twice a day on an empty stomach, is known to promptly cure oral and pharyngeal thrush. Esophageal candida infections, in which the infection may spread toward the lungs, require a physician's immediate attention. With a cost of about sixty-five cents per day, regular use of Pau D'Arco is possibly useful as a prophylaxis against more serious systemic fungal infections.

Garlic

Known to be one of the most potent antimicrobial agents ever discovered, Albert Schweitzer used garlic to treat amoebic dysentery and Louis Pasteur used it as an antibacterial. Garlic has been shown to be effective against all but two of twenty-six strains of candida albicans. In the March 1985 issue of *Scientific American,* it was reported that garlic was effective against 200 varieties of pathogenic fungi.[13]

Garlic is also one of the richest sources of the element germanium, known to be a potent inducer of interferon. Germanium has also shown effectiveness against certain types of cancers by modulating the immune response.

Garlic can be used to treat candida infections by taking gelatin capsules filled with fresh minced garlic. Up to two cloves a day may be required for serious infections. Fresh garlic is generally considered to be far superior to the extracts and dried products on health food store shelves. Taken concomitantly, parsley and fennel offset garlic's strong odor. Garlic is also known to be effective for treating intestinal parasites and some bacterial infections. Its broad spectrum of use and its low cost—thirty cents per day—make the "Stinking Rose" an attractive method for treating candida infection.

Gamma-Linoleic Acid (GLA)

GLA is an essential fatty acid often extracted from evening primrose flowers. It is also found in cold-pressed olive, linseed, sesame, and borage seed oils. Consuming more GLA helps prevent candida from becoming systematically invasive. GLA is also known to have other beneficial effects on immune regulation.

Lactobacillus

A group of friendly microorganisms that transform milk into yogurt and cheese, lactobacillus are useful in helping maintain the delicate balance of fungus and bacteria in the intestinal tract. Some good brands are Jarrowdophilus, Primadophilus, and Megadophilus. Using these products is reported to gradually reverse mucocutaneous fungal infections.

Tea Tree Oil

This extract of a tree native to Australia is a tried-and-true remedy for many mucosal fungal infections. The oil is diluted in water (six drops per four ounces of water) and gargled, allowing it to reach deep into the back of the throat. It tastes terrible, but it works, usually in just one or two doses. It can also be applied in diluted form to fungal skin and nailbed infections. Tea Tree Oil is cheap and widely available in health food stores.

Biotin

Biotin is a B-vitamin essential for the metabolism of fats and proteins. It is believed to play a role in preventing candida from converting into its invasive form. Available in supplement form, Biotin is fairly inexpensive. 5 to 10 mg. are reported as useful doses for treating thrush infections.

Dietary Interventions

Diet lays an important role in keeping indigenous flora in check. Fungus, particularly yeasts like candida, thrive on sugar and overprocessed carbohydrates. Decreasing your consumption of foods containing these ingredients can help keep this nuisance to a minimum.

Immune Modulating Nutrients: Vitamin A and Zinc (9/17/92)

A commonly held misconception is that a well balanced-diet will meet all of our nutritional needs. However, the modern diet is replete with processed foods having diminished nutrient composition, and other factors, such as the body's ability to absorb nutrients, must also be considered.

In fact, malnutrition is the most common cause of immunodeficiency worldwide. Many people with AIDS-related illness have complex health factors inhibiting their bodies' absorption of vitamins and minerals. Supplementation to maintain adequate levels may be required to insulate the intact elements of the immune system from further damage.

Several studies on immune modulating properties were discussed at the 1992 Amsterdam AIDS Conference. In this article, I will discuss two essential nutrients and the role they play in human immunology: Vitamin A and Zinc.[14]

Vitamin A

Discovered over fifty years ago, Retinol, known as vitamin A, was originally classified as an anti-infective agent. It plays an important role in rapidly renewing tissues associated with growth, reproduction, and bone formation. Vitamin A deficiency is often associated with protein-energy malnutrition. It is a fat-soluble vitamin and can be toxic at high doses.

Vitamin A was first seen as an immunomodulator as a result of the observation that susceptibility to infection and the development of tumors in vitamin A-deficient human subjects was easily and quickly reversed by replenishment of the vitamin. Based on this, it is believed that vitamin A can, at nontoxic doses, act as an adjuvant, or enhancing agent, of the immune response.

Vitamin A deficiency is now associated with the suppression of both the innate and acquired branches of the immune system. While the function of vitamin A in immunology is not clearly understood at this time, it is known that loss of cellular integrity caused by inadequate vitamin A results in adverse consequences to individuals' immunity. Examples of negative effects are reduced antibody production and increased susceptibility of tissues to the adherence of pathogenic organisms.

Circumstantial evidence suggests that vitamin A stimulates the bactericidal activities of several specialized white blood cells, particularly macrophages and natural killers. It is known to enhance the delayed-type hypersensitivity reaction, a good indicator of cell-mediated immune functioning.

Vitamin A deficiency also adversely affects the lymphoid system. The thymus gland and bone marrow, where T-lymphocytes are generated, mature, and differentiate, develop atrophy and lose mass due to deficiency of this vitamin. In animal studies, T-cell subsets were 60 percent lower in vitamin A-deficient mice than in the control group fed adequate amounts of the vitamin.

All impairments caused by deficiency of vitamin A can be reversed by adequate supplementation. But vitamin A in its most commonly used form is toxic at high doses, and should not be consumed in daily doses exceeding ten mg. Deficiencies can occur even in cases of adequate dietary intake, particularly in the presence of abnormalities of fat ingestion and absorption, such as intestinal infections, which are extremely common among people with AIDS. The vitamin tends to accumulate in the liver, and requires zinc to release it in the bloodstream where it has its most therapeutic action.

Beta carotene is a nontoxic substance that can be stored in the body and converted into vitamin A by the liver as needed. A naturally occurring plant product (it is the agent that imparts red and yellow pigment to certain vegetables), beta carotene, or provitamin A, is the chemical precursor of vitamin A. Nontoxic even at high doses, it ensures avoidance of vitamin A deficiency. Suggested dose is 25,000 I.U. per day, but some immune-compromised people use up to 50,000 I.U. per day. Beta carotene is also known to function as an anti-oxidant and scavenger of damaging free radicals of oxygen, helping to protect the body from certain carcinogens and possibly viruses.

Zinc

An essential trace nutrient, zinc is critical to the functioning of the immune system and is also needed for the optimal use of vitamin A. Yet zinc deficiency is very common, and this condition is clearly recognized in medicine as a critical factor in chronic disease.

Some effects of zinc deficiency on immune competence include T-lymphocyte dysfunction and atrophy of the thymus gland, where T-cells are produced. Cell-mediated immunity is also impeded by zinc deficiency, resulting in anergic delayed-type hypersensitivity. Lack of zinc can result in diminished T-cell dependent antibodies, decreased populations of cells in the monocyte/macrophage system, and lower levels of Interleukin-2, a cytokine that signals the growth and differentiation of T-lymphocytes.

Zinc deficiency causes wounds to heal more slowly, which is why zinc oxide is commonly used as a topical healing agent. Natural killer cell activity appears to be inhibited by zinc insufficiency, and individuals with inadequate zinc supply are more susceptible to infectious diseases and suffer more severely from them. Zinc's function of facilitating the transport of vitamin A from the liver to other parts of the body is critical. Without zinc, vitamin A deficiency can occur even in the presence of an adequate dietary supply of the vitamin.

Zinc is not absorbed well by those who eat a high fiber diet. Supplements, which are inexpensive, should be labeled as containing "amino acid chelating agents" or "transport complexers" in order to maximize the body's use of zinc. Fifteen mg. is the Recommended Dietary Allowance (RDA), but many people consume from sixty to 100 mg. per day to assure adequate levels. Zinc appears to be non-toxic at these dosages.

Maintaining adequate levels of Vitamin A and Zinc is clearly essential for the immune system to function normally. Assuring that the body has all the raw material it needs to enhance its own healing systems is especially important for people living with HIV. Proper nutrient supplementation is a good way to contribute to the body's natural disease fighting abilities.

Germanium: Potent Immune Modulator from Japan (10/1/92)

The mineral Germanium, with an atomic weight of thirty-two on the periodic table of elements, is not known to be essential to human health. Yet considerable research into its therapeutic effects on the immune system is underway in several countries, including the United States and Japan.[15]

Discovered in 1886, Germanium was initially thought to be rare and received little attention until its unique property of conductivity was discovered. This discovery ultimately had profound effects on the development of computer technology and led to its use as the conductor in the first transistor. Germanium was later used in Texas Instrument's development of the first microchip, prior to the use of silicon.

Kuzihiko Asai, a Japanese geologist, discovered that coal deposits, which are fossilized plants, contain Germanium. Asai extracted a crystalline, water-soluble, highly stable organic compound which he called bis-carboxethyl Germanium sesquioxide, or GE-132. While very little of it exists naturally in the earth's crust, it is now known that the mineral concentrates in plants. In the 1960s, Japanese researchers founded the Asai Germanium Research Institute to formally undertake studies studies of the mineral's effects on animal and human biology. Medically-supervised studies of Germanium in human physiology are currently in progress at twenty-seven Japanese institutions.

In the United States, the Germanium Institute of North America, a cooperative organization that is now defunct, operated for several years under the supervision of biochemist Stephen Levine, Ph.D. Dr. Levine claims that his research has shown that Germanium is at the same time a profound immunostimulant, an oxygen facilitator, and a blocker of free radicals of oxygen. He also claims that organic Germanium is a dramatic immune modulator with antitumor effects and interferon inducing activities.[16] Additionally, Germanium has been reported to restore immune function in immunodepressed animals.[17]

Beside inducing interferon production, researchers believe Germanium induces the production of Tumor Necrosis Factor-alpha (TNF-α), which would help to explain its antitumor properties. It is also believed to increase production of these immunologic substances by direct stimulation of the monocyte/macrophage system. Germanium is known to increase the numbers and activity of natural killer cells and researchers speculate that it has some direct antiviral activity. Germanium may normalize the function of T-lymphocytes, B-lymphocytes, and antibody-dependent cellular cytotoxicity (ADCC).[18]

Germanium also decreases food intolerances, although the way it does so is unknown. It also has analgesic properties; one gram of Germanium can immediately stop intractable cancer pain and is commonly used in Japan as an adjuvant to cancer chemotherapy and radiation therapy. It helps regulate all body systems in postsurgical cases and keep white blood counts within normal ranges, for which it is used medically in Japanese surgical hospitals.

Notably, holistic practitioners consider the richest sources of organic Germanium to be medicinal plants. At this point, the role Germanium plays in the medicinal qualities of such plants as garlic, aloe vera, ginseng, barley, and chlorella can only be speculated.

No certain immunomodulating dose is recommended. Only products labeled GE-132 or Ge-Oxy are the correct preparations. As Germanium is not absorbed well through the gastrointestinal tract, Dr. Levine recommends small sublingual doses throughout the course of the day, with a maximum dose of 150 mg. four times a day. Most people use about one-quarter to one-half that amount.

It is available in powdered form at better health food retailers or buyer's clubs. A five gram bottle should cost no more than twenty dollars. Both GE-132 and Ge-Oxy are believed to be very stable and nontoxic. However, toxic side effects such as renal impairment have been attributed to the use of Germanium in nonstabilized form. Some people have reported that the use of Germanium stimulates the central nervous system and recommend that it be taken in the morning so as not to interfere with sleep.

Germanium is yet another naturally-occurring and apparently safe substance that has eluded the interest of the Western medical establishment. Few references to it appear in the conventional medical literature, but enough is known about it to warrant a closer examination by those who feel that it may be beneficial to them.

Vitamin C and Immunity
(10/15/92)

One of the most universally common factors in the health regimen of long-term AIDS survivors is their increased consumption of vitamin C. Few nutrients are as biologically active in human metabolism as ascorbic acid, known to be the most important water-soluble antioxidant and cofactor in cellular metabolism. Several researchers have clearly demonstrated that the immune system is sensitive to the intake levels of vitamin C.

The Encyclopedia of Immunology includes a chapter on "Vitamin C and the Immune System," in which numerous immunological functions dependent on vitamin C for their mediation are identified.[19] The correlation between decreases in vitamin C intake and decreased immunity and susceptibility to infections has been clearly proven. Vitamin C is known to induce the production of interferon and to have some direct antimicrobial effect. Part of its antimicrobial property lies in its ability to inhibit replication of viruses. Carefully designed, placebo-controlled double blind human studies have shown that vitamin C not only lessened the severity of the rhinovirus cold, but also reduced the risk of person-to-person infection.

Vitamin C is essential to the antioxidant free radical scavenging functions of the immune system, achieved by protecting the antioxidant properties of vitamin E, a potent immune enhancing nutrient in its own right. Other important functions include enhanced cell-mediated immunity, as demonstrated by improved delayed-type hypersensitivity. This vitamin is necessary for the activation of white blood cells for bactericidal activity, and protects white cells from a process called auto-oxidation that compromises cellular antibacterial activity.

Human beings are among the few animal species who do not possess the capacity to synthesize vitamin C, making sufficient dietary intake of the vitamin necessary to health. Some people with chronic illness opt to use extremely high doses of this vitamin in the belief that its virucidal and immunomodulating properties will be maximized by keeping body tissue saturated with a therapeutic level of the nutrient. Since vitamin C is water soluble, it is believed that continual dose replenishment is needed, especially during times of illness, as it is continually flushed out of the body. Therapeutic dosages used by many PWAs to achieve the necessary levels go as high as twenty grams per day. Generally, the dose is gradually increased over time until the development of gastrointestinal discomfort, at which time dosage decreased gradually until the side effects abate.

Concerning the at times extreme anecdotal medical claims for vitamin C, it is often difficult to tell fact from fiction. But sufficient numbers of serious laboratory investigations and animal and human studies have found that maintenance of adequate, steady levels of this critical nutrient help maintain the functioning and integrity of many parts of the immune system. Vitamin C can be purchased in tablet, capsule, or powdered form. If ingesting vitamin C powder dissolved in water or juice, drink with a straw— ascorbic acid can, over time, erode tooth enamel. Studies indicate that the optimal amount of vitamin C is two to three grams per day. Greater amounts can cause possible immunosuppression.[20]

An inexpensive nutrient with known antiviral, immunomodulating, and antioxidant properties, vitamin C would appear a likely candidate for dietary supplementation, particularly in immune-suppressed individuals and those suffering from other degenerative illnesses. Many healthy PWAs, too many to ignore, swear by it.

Chinese Medicine and HIV Disease
(12/3/92)

Acupuncture and Chinese herbal medications have become some of the most commonly used alternative therapies for AIDS in the Bay

Area. In fact, their use have become so widely accepted that two Chinese Medicine clinics in San Francisco have been awarded contracts through the San Francisco Health Department, AIDS Office to provide Chinese Medical treatment to people with HIV. The contracts are funded by the Ryan White CARE Act allocations.

Most people with HIV who use acupuncture and Chinese herbs do so in conjunction with Western medicine. There are, however, some who use it as their principal form of medical treatment. In any case, it is strongly suggested that it be used under the supervision of a licensed practitioner. In California, the practice of Traditional Chinese Medicine (TCM) is considered a primary care medical modality and its practitioners are regarded as physicians. Certain components of TCM practice are reimbursable by private insurance companies. For example, acupuncture is covered by Medi-CAL at a rate of two treatments per month. Practitioners of Chinese Medicine are titled Licensed Acupuncturists, or L.Ac., and are licensed by the State Board of Medical Quality Assurance. Rigorous training is required to qualify to sit for the licensing examination, including three years of postgraduate training in Chinese Medicine, with additional training in Western-based anatomy, physiology, and biology.

According to Natural Healing with Chinese Herbs by Dr. Hong-yen Hsu, Ph.D., the systematic practice of Chinese Medicine dates back over two thousand years, making it the oldest medical system in the world. The first known medical book on the subject is The Yellow Emperor's Classic of Internal Medicine, written during the Han Dynasty, around 200 B.C.E. The Treatise on Febrile Diseases, the first systematic compendium of collected knowledge on the subject, appeared at approximately the same time. Its author, Chang Chung-ching, is considered historically to be among China's greatest physicians; he is as revered in China as is Hippocrates in the West. From its very origins, Chinese Medicine combined empirical experience with a clear philosophical theory.

Many people erroneously view Chinese herbal praxis as a rough equivalent to the Western practice of taking a drug for the alleviation of symptoms. However, there are profound differences between the two approaches. Where Western medicine is derived solely from scientific method of treating disease, Chinese medicine stems from a philosophical foundation based on a holistic view of supporting the mind-body's innate ability to maintain health and to heal itself should illness occur. Chinese medicine is the result of many thousands of years of accumulated experience and wisdom.

Chinese philosophy views the universe as a living organism and sees the human body as a microcosm of that larger organism. In contrast, Western medicine tends to view the human body mechanistically and has evolved its practice based on the assumption that the body is a machine with essentially separate but linked components. Rather than dealing only with discrete components of the human organism, as Western science advocates, the TCM approach is one of aligning the functions of the organs and internal systems as a whole, promoting the dynamic balance of energy polarities crucial to good health and well-being.

Central to Chinese medical philosophy is the concept of *ch'i,* or *qi,* loosely defined as the vital energy of the universe from which all things derive. Ch'i patterns fluctuate between polarities of yin and yang, the active and passive sides of the life force. Chinese medicine views illness as either an excess or deficiency in either the yin or yang components of ch'i.

Ch'i is believed to vitalize the body as it moves along its internal pathways, known as meridians. Because Western medicine has not been able to objectively identify the anatomical location of these pathways, the "meridian theory" of Chinese medicine is not accepted. For Chinese doctors, however, circumstantial evidence of their existence is undeniable. Points along the meridians have been used successfully as acupuncture sites for thousands of years. Herbs are also thought to facilitate the normal movement of ch'i along the meridians. The Japanese term for illness, *bioki,* translates as "injured ch'i." Dr. Gonzon Goto, a leading Japanese authority on Chinese medicine, contends that the cause of all disease is the obstruction of ch'i along the meridians.

In San Francisco, Misha Cohen, a Doctor of Oriental Medicine, popularized Chinese medicine as a treatment for AIDS beginning in 1984. Much Western research on certain aspects of Chinese Medicine has since been conducted. Many herbs used in Chinese medicine have been found to inhibit HIV and other viruses in laboratory experiments while others have been shown to act as biological response modifiers, enhancing certain immune responses. In addition, in a small, strictly-controlled study conducted at Lincoln Hospital, New York in the mid-80s, individuals receiving correctly applied acupuncture had notable increases in their CD4 counts after only a brief course of therapy. This pilot study certainly demonstrated the need for further research into acupuncture therapy for HIV.

The most attractive feature of Chinese medicine is its complete lack of toxicity when administered by trained professionals. People should not use Chinese herbal formulations without the supervision of a licensed practitioner of TCM. Herbs can be obtained in various forms, and are relatively inexpensive. Take special care with herbs that increase antibodies, as their use can result in suppression of cellular immunity.[21] Several human efficacy studies of Chinese medicine for HIV disease are currently underway or enrolling participants under the supervision of the FDA. Chinese herbs may be a rich source of therapeutic agents for AIDS and its related illnesses and their properties and use are well worth looking into.

Cellular and Antibody Immune Responses in AIDS
(4/8/93)
Billi Goldberg

At the dawning of the Age of AIDS, scientists had a very simplistic view of the immune system: antibodies, antibodies, and more antibodies. Now they are finding that the human immune system is much more complicated than they previously imagined. Most people are familiar with antibodies and believe that they provide protection against the opportunistic infections in AIDS. That, simply put, is not true. It is now known that production of antibodies, or humoral immunity, enables viral and other microbial pathogens to flourish because it does not destroy the infected cells that are the source of infection, but only temporarily controls cell-free or cell-surface infectious microbes.

The other arm of the immune system, cell-mediated immunity (CMI), or cellular immunity, is critical in controlling and clearing the infectious agents that cause opportunistic diseases in AIDS.[22] The primary effector cells in CMI are activated macrophages, natural killer (NK) cells and cytotoxic T-lymphocytes. It is the natural function of these cells to destroy all infected and abnormal cells, including HIV-infected CD4 cells.[23] These effector cells are activated by delayed-type hypersensitivity (DTH), which is a form of cell-mediated immunity using CD4 cells.

Flu, colds, and many common viral and other infections are controlled by humoral immunity which will clear the cell-free or cell-surface (extracellular, exogenous) pathogens. Cellular infection is not a problem in these infections because the cells infected by these pathogens are continually being destroyed and replaced. Thus, there are no long-lived cells to continue to spread infectious matter. HIV and the opportunistic infections and neoplasms seen in AIDS are considered as being *in* the cells (intracellular, endogenous) and can only be controlled by cellular immunity initiated by delayed-type hypersensitivity.[24] The defective cellular immunity (and not a defect of humoral/antibody immunity) was the first recognized hallmark of AIDS in 1981, and this continues to be the cause of disease progression.

There are two types of CD4 cells. The first, Th1, initiates delayed-type hypersensitivity which invokes cellular immunity. The CD8 cells activated by Th1 are known as T1. Th2, the second type of CD4 cell, initiates antibody responses. The CD8 cells in this Th2 response suppress cellular immunity and are known as T2.[25] The critical aspect is that opportunistic infections and HIV in AIDS are considered to be *in the cells* and thus can only be controlled by cellular immunity (Th1/T1).

CD4 cells are inadequate for determining immune system status because they can be either Th1 (good) or Th2 (bad). The CD8 cytotoxic subset (T1) is more predictive of immune system responsiveness to opportunistic infections. In actuality, high absolute numbers of CD8 cells (500 and above) are generally indicative of probable long-term survival. Systemic activation of Th1 will suppress Th2 and, conversely, activation of Th2 will suppress Th1. All of these immune responses are controlled by cytokines.[26] In the Th1 response, IL-2 and IFN-gamma predominate; in the Th2 response, IL-4 and IL-10 predominate.[27]

Scientists at the National Cancer Institute have recently discov-

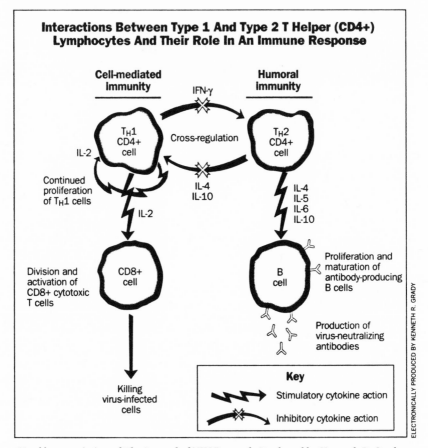

Used by permission of *The Journal of NIH Research*. Produced by Kenneth R. Grady

ered that in HIV infection, a switch from Th1 (cellular immunity) to a predominance of Th2 (humoral immunity) is an indicator of disease progression from the asymptomatic stage into full-blown AIDS.[28] The researchers concluded that the opportunistic infections (viral, bacterial, fungal, parasitic) and neoplasms seen in AIDS, including HIV, flourish when cellular immunity (Th1) is suppressed and humoral immunity (Th2) is dominant. They also believe that an imbalance between Th1 and Th2, with Th2 dominant, may actually predispose individuals to HIV infection.[29]

Successful treatments and vaccines for AIDS must therefore be able to stimulate cellular immunity (Th1/T1 response) and suppress humoral immunity (Th2/T2 response).[30] Stimulation of cellular immunity, *not* stimulation of antibodies or suppression of the immune system, will probably be the only way that HIV infection will become a chronic, rather than fatal, disease.[31] Most of the approved treatments and prophylaxis for HIV and opportunistic infections are immunosuppressive and must be used judiciously as they impair cellular immunity. Notably, most individuals who have AIDS are fully capable of controlling infections that rely on the humoral or antibody response, but are incapable of controlling infections that depend on cellular immunity.

End Game, or How HIV Causes AIDS
(5/12/93)
Billi Goldberg

How HIV infection causes AIDS is slowly but surely being understood and explained. And, surprise, surprise—it is not because HIV infects CD4 cells. Another sacred pronouncement of establishment scientists and researchers is falling by the wayside. The consistency of their errors in the pathogenesis of AIDS is remarkable: wrong, 100 percent of the time!

AIDS is not caused by depletion of CD4 cells. It is caused by HIV infection, dysfunction, and the ultimate destruction of the cells that present the intracellular microbes (virus, bacteria, fungi, and protozoa) that cause opportunistic infections to the CD4 and CD8 cells.[32] When infected, these antigen-presenting cells can no longer appropriately activate CD4 and CD8 cells to begin to proliferate and form additional helper, effector, and memory cells.[33] The end result of this continual decrease in the total number of T-lymphocytes is an impaired immune response and progression to full-blown AIDS.[34]

Dendritic cells, Langerhans cells, macrophages, and B-cells are the primary antigen-presenting cells in the immune system.[35] Each of these, except B-cells, are capable of being infected by HIV. B-cells, the precursors of antibody-forming cells, are crucial in the formation of the antibody or Th2 response. The antibody response in HIV-positive individuals is, for the most part, not impaired in HIV/AIDS except for being overactive. The immune system is still capable of activating the subset of CD4 cells that are used in initiating an antibody (Th2) response.

Recent research indicates that dendritic cells are the most efficient antigen-presenting cells (APC) in the immune system.[36] In 1993, researchers stated that dendritic cells, when infected with HIV, could not present antigen to CD4 and CD8 cells in such a way that they would be activated and could proliferate.[37] This dysfunction (anergy) results from the inability of these APCs to provide the co-stimulatory signal required to initiate the cell-mediated (Th1) immune response.[38] This response includes cytotoxic T-lymphocytes, which are required to destroy infected cells. If this is not accomplished, infected cells continue to be reservoirs of various infections, such as HIV and the other microbes that cause the opportunistic infections seen in AIDS.[39]

Even though these dysfunctional antigen-presenting cells cannot cause proliferation of cytotoxic T-lymphocytes, they are still destroyed by the CD8 cells, because the CD8 cells are still cytolytic or destructive even when anergic.[40] The decreased number of antigen-presenting cells in AIDS progression is an established fact that has been exhaustingly documented in the scientific literature.[41]

A study published earlier this year shows that the Epstein-Barr virus (EBV) is still capable of activating cytotoxic T-lymphocytes even in the latter stages of AIDS. Interestingly, B-cells are the antigen-presenting cells for EBV infection, and they are not infected by HIV. The authors also showed that HIV-infected macrophages in the same individuals were increasingly unable to activate HIV-specific cytotoxic T-lymphocytes during progression of HIV infection.[42]

The result of this deficiency in activating CD8 cells is a constantly decreasing number of total CD8 cells and, hence, an increase in viral replication.[43] As viral replication increases, so does the number of HIV dysfunctional antigen-presenting cells, leading to an ever-increasing number of opportunistic infections. If the infected antigen-presenting cells cannot present HIV, they surely cannot present the infectious virus, bacteria, fungi, and protozoa that cause opportunistic infections.[44]

Finally, research published just this month puts the icing on the cake. The authors explain that T-cell dysfunction in HIV infection is undoubtedly due to anergy caused by defective antigen-presenting cells in a succinct statement: "Alteration of the functions of the antigen-presenting cell may program T-cells for activation-induced death, and may induce anergy in interleukin-2 and interferon-gamma secreting TH1 cells. This results in predominance of TH2 allergic response instead of cellular immunity dependent on TH1 cells."[45]

The article goes on to say, "HIV-infected chimpanzees do not develop HIV-related disease and evidence for PCD [programmed cell death] and significant defects in T-cell function are not found. Interestingly, HIV does not infect monocytes from chimpanzees and only T-cell tropic variants are isolated from infected animals." Now, here is a logical and elegant explanation for why the "experts" have never been able to find an animal model for HIV/AIDS, forcing them to rely on human guinea pigs. Driving this point home emphatically, the article powerfully and simply states, "The absence of infected APC [antigen-presenting cells] in chimpanzees strengthens the importance of infection of APC for the induction of immunodeficiency and AIDS-like disease."

If the Th1 or cellular immunity is incapable of being activated, the microbes that cause opportunistic infections will thrive and flourish, resulting in damage to vital organs and progression to the AIDS endpoint: death. Immunosuppressing prophylaxis drugs appear to speed this progression by interfering with what is left of the immune system's ability to respond to various infections. Vaccines[46] and other treatments that enhance antibody or Th2 responses shut down cellular immunity, resulting in increased opportunistic infections.

The end game for HIV/AIDS is now being played out. The cause of AIDS is not HIV acting alone, but acting indirectly by infection of the primary antigen-presenting cells of the cellular immune system: dendritic cells, Langerhans cells, and macrophages. Perhaps now, the "experts" will focus on immunotherapies to boost the cellular immune system and destroy infected cells. The bone marrow will then replace destroyed cells with new cells that are not infected. Of course, this is dependent on a bone marrow that has not been destroyed by drug toxicity or infection from longstanding immunosuppression. For too long, research efforts have concentrated on treatments that depress the immune system, cause horrendous side effects, and result in nothing but suffering and death for tens of thousands of people infected with HIV.

The "experts" have been wrong about CD4 cells being a meaningful surrogate marker; they have been wrong about the percentage of CD4 cells that are infected with HIV; they have been wrong about antiretroviral treatments; and they have been wrong about the so-called latency period of HIV replication. Is it any big surprise, then, that they have been wrong about HIV infection of CD4 cells causing AIDS?

Macrophage Activation by Direct Stimulation (5/26/93)
Charles R. Caulfield and Billi Goldberg

Scientists involved in AIDS and related research have spent billions of dollars and millions of research hours trying to stimulate the immune system to respond to cancer, viral infections, and the microbial pathogens that cause opportunistic infections. Their focus has been on naturally-occurring cytokines (soluble intercellular signaling molecules) that the body produces to control the primary cell-mediated (Th1), antibody (Th2), and inflammatory immune responses.

With great hubris, medical establishment "experts" have been learning how to produce these cytokines utilizing recombinant technology and synthetic peptides in a fruitless quest for the "magic bullet" that will cure human ills and repair the toxic effects of the nucleoside analogues, cancer treatments, and antibiotic drugs. Conversely, they have also investigated the process of impeding immune system production of some cytokines because they have, in their wisdom, decided that too much of a specific cytokine is bad.

Rather than adopting a holistic perspective on the immune system, which is comprised of many interdependent components, scientific research is attempting to dissect the immune system and deal with its discrete components as if they existed in a vacuum. This minimalist approach cannot possibly succeed at any meaningful level; for molecular biologists specifically, it has not succeeded to any meaningful degree in a forty-year quest for successful gene therapies.

The key to successfully invoking both systemic and localized immune responses lies in the use of exogenous biological response modifiers that are nontoxic, inexpensive, and capable of activation without interfering with the natural production of cytokines. DNCB has shown positive results in activating a systemic Th1 response; Acemannan is now showing promise by activating localized immune responses that originate with macrophages. DNCB and Acemannan are the only two therapies that have a demonstrated ability to activate cytotoxic T-lymphocytes and natural killer cells capable of destroying infected cells.[47] Acemannan has already been USDA-approved for the treatment of cancers and retroviral infections in animals, and it has also been used to treat human cancers with some positive results.[48]

Macrophages are a key element in unlocking the mysteries of AIDS and controlling intracellular infections. They originate in the bone marrow and enter the circulation as monocytes. In less than a day, they leave circulation, differentiate into macrophages, and enter tissues. An adult's body contain billions of monocytes and macrophages. If infected with HIV, these white blood cells can spread the infection to all parts of the body when entering the tissues.[49] They reside in the liver, brain, spleen, lymph nodes, bone marrow, thymus, nerves, lungs, bones, and elsewhere in the body, and are critical to normal immune functioning in these areas. Macrophages are the body's scavengers: they internalize and destroy foreign bodies such as damaged cells and infectious microorganisms in a process known as phagocytosis.

Macrophages are the potential reservoirs of a host of infections, including HSV, CMV, HIV, Chlamydia, Mycobacteria (TB, MAI, MAC), Salmonella, Aspergillus, Candida, Cryptococcus, Histoplasma, Toxoplasma, and Leishmania.[50] Not only do they present antigen to cytotoxic and helper T-lymphocytes, but macrophages are lethal both to microbes and tumors through various means, including reactive oxygen intermediates (ROI) and secretion of tumor necrosis factors (TNF). However, in their natural state as a resting cell, macrophages are of little value in presenting antigen, secreting TNF, destroying microbes, or killing tumor cells. If macrophages can be properly primed and activated, they can accomplish the critical functions required to control infections and tumor cells.

To activate the immune system locally, Interleukin-1 must be secreted from macrophages or Interferon-gamma from T-lymphocytes. In healthy immune systems, these secretions are accomplished without problem. The end result is not only activation and proliferation of T-lymphocytes, but upregulation of macrophages to their primed and activated states. In HIV/AIDS individuals, this process becomes increasingly less efficient as the disease progresses and interferes with the ability of HIV-infected antigen-presenting cells to initiate immune responses. An especially interesting fact about macrophages is that their activation results in a down-regulation of HIV production in HIV-infected macrophages, just the opposite of the reported increase in HIV replication in activated HIV-infected CD4 cells.[51]

With weekly injections, Acemannan appears to be rendered capable of entering dormant macrophages residing in tissues through their mannose receptors. After processing, this results in the production of Interleukin-1 (IL-1), Interleukin-6 (IL-6), and Tumor Necrosis Factor (TNF).[52] IL-1, with IL-6 as a costimulator, can stimulate cytotoxic and helper T-lymphocytes to produce appropriate cytokines, primarily Interferon-gamma, which in turn initiates cell-mediated immune responses and activates macrophages.[53] IL-1 and IL-6 secretions have the added benefit of stimulating the production of factors that result in increased bone-marrow production of important white blood cells (such as neutrophils). Acemannan, therefore, can directly stimulate macrophages to their primed and activated states.

Those who respond to Acemannan indicate activation of their cellular immunity, resulting in increased control of opportunistic infections and halting of disease progression for a few years. Since only 20 to 40 percent of Acemannan users respond to the drug, the treatment has never attained widespread acceptance as an HIV/AIDS therapy. Possible reasons for nonresponse are that no drug can access only infected cells; or that the drug activates antibody responses (Th2) by the IL-1 and IL-6 secretions.

Since Acemannan activates the macrophages it enters, it could be a valuable tool in triggering destruction of intracellular microbes (virus, bacteria, fungi and protozoa) that cause opportunistic infections in AIDS. The key to Acemannan efficacy is to control the type

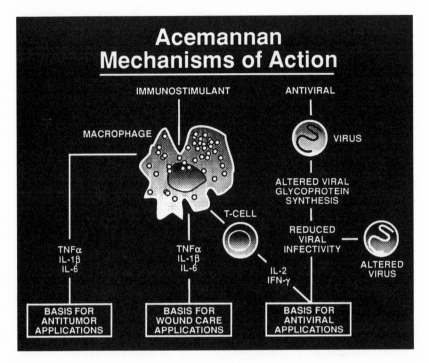

Used by permission of Carrington Laboratories.

of immune response it initiates. In preliminary testing, it appears that combining DNCB with injectable Acemannan might just result in the synergism required for a salvage treatment for those with low CD4s and CD8s, along with breakouts of opportunistic infections. DNCB has never been considered a salvage therapy for severely immunosuppressed individuals.

The premise for this treatment strategy is that those who do not respond to Acemannan have initiated an antibody (Th2) rather than a cell-mediated response (Th1), a reasonable explanation as both IL-1 and IL-6 have the ability to augment B-cell activation and antibody production. Since DNCB invokes a Th1 systemic response,[54] it would then shut down the Th2 response initiated by Acemannan, thus greatly increasing the number of responders to Acemannan. DNCB, when initiating the systemic Th1 response, could activate infected macrophages that were not stimulated by Acemannan.

101

When used as a salvage therapy for a few months (after DNCB sensitization), Acemannan would cost less than twenty dollars per month. Once the disease progression is halted and individuals have been stabilized, they would continue to use DNCB alone as a pro-phylaxis, resulting in an even lower-cost treatment regimen. A phase I trial of injectable Acemannan has not shown any toxicity in much higher doses than proposed for the combination treatment with DNCB. As has become the norm in the quest for successful HIV/AIDS therapies, both underground and "sanctioned" trials are now taking place under the supervision of alternative treatment physicians and knowledgeable activists.

How DNCB Works
Billi Goldberg

DNCB, applied in weekly applications on the skin, initiates contact sensitivity. The Langerhans cells in the skin at the application site pick up the DNCB antigen, migrate from the skin, change into veiled dendritic cells, continue their migration to the nearest lymph node, and change into interdigitating dendritic cells. Once in the lymph nodes, they present the DNCB antigen to CD4 helper cells, initiating what is called alternately a Th1 response, cell-mediated immune response, or Type IV Delayed-type hypersensitivity response.

The CD4 helper cells proliferate forming more helper CD4 cells which then circulate and activate effector cells (primarily macrophages) to rid the sysem of the DNCB antigen. At the same time, CD4 memory cells are produced, adding to the CD4 memory pool for the DNCB antigen (hapten). Each time DNCB is applied, these memory cells are activated, thus initiating a systemic Th1 response to DNCB. The longer DNCB is used, the faster, more potent, and more effective the response becomes, as there are more circu-lating DNCB CD4 memory cells to initiate the immune response.

The result of this specific systemic Th1 response to DNCB is the nonspecific activation of macrophages. Many of these macrophages are infected with HIV and other intracellular pathogens that cause AIDS but are unable to present these pathogen antigens due to infection. The microbial pathogens of AIDS are of the facultative or obligate intracellular type. The activation of these macrophages result in proteolysis of the pathogens which are then presented by macrophages to CD4 and CD8 memory cells specific for the presented pathogen. The activated helper and cytotoxic T-lymphocytes initiate specific systemic responses to destroy the presented pathogens. This results in more activated macrophages, more pathogens presented, more T-memory cells activated, more infected cells destroyed, ad infinitum.

Since pathogens can be presented on both the Class I and Class II MHC (major histocompatibility complex) of the antigen-presenting cells, cytotoxic T-lymphocytes, natural killer cells, neutrophils, and killer macrophages are also activated to accomplish the destruction. There is also excellent probability that dendritic cells (the most potent antigen-presenting cells in the immune system) are also activated in the lymphoid tissues to present intracellular and extracellular antigens, thereby activating even more T-lymphocyte memory, helper, and effector cells and increasing the Th1 response against the pathogens involved in AIDS.

It is extremely important to remember that the antibody/Th2/ humoral response is not directly involved in fighting AIDS-related infections. Denial of this fact is the primary reason there has been no progress in realistic treatments for AIDS. In point of fact, there is research showing that activating the antibody or Th2 response may suppress the Th1 response. This would allow the intracellular pathogens to be uncontrolled, since their control depends on the Th1 or cell-mediated immune response. There is also research indicating that immune complexes (HIV + antibody) can be internalized through the antibody receptor (Fc) of monocytes and macrophages, thus spreading and increasing HIV infection of these cells.[55]

Delayed-Type Hypersensitivity is an extremely effective and potent immune modulator that forces the priming and activation of macrophages that are nonresponsive due to infection. DNCB, then, acts as an adjuvant or biological response modifier. These phenomena have been researched in depth and are considered a factual part of scientific knowledge.[56] DNCB has also been used for years in delayed hypersensitivity skin tests.[57]

The process by which DNCB works has been an integral part of the scientific literature for many years. DNCB is not new; it has been used for decades. But, as we have noted previously, the minimal cost of DNCB makes it an unlikely candidate for further research as there is no profit to be made. Following are excerpts from "Delayed-type Hypersensitivity and the Induction of Activated, Cytotoxic Macrophages" by Monte S. Meltzer and Carol A. Nacy, from *Fundamental Immunology*.

"Contact sensitivity is a variant form of DTH in which certain reactive chemicals (usually small molecular weight compounds or metal ions that can diffuse into the epidermis) covalently bind to skin proteins and create neoantigens. Such neoantigens prime or sensitize the exposed animal to a second cutaneous application of the reactive chemical (contactant). A portion of the neoantigen is host derived. Thus an animal exposed to trinitrochlorobenzene (TNCB or picryl chloride) solution epicutaneously responds to a repeated cutaneous exposure with a vigorous DTH response. Intradermal injection of TNCB covalently bound to an irrelevant protein such as albumin fails to elicit this response. Neoantigens induced in the epidermis are taken up by Langerhans cells. These highly efficient, antigen-presenting dendritic cells migrate into the dermis, enter lymphatics, and travel to the cortical region of the draining lymph node where they present the antigen to CD4+ T-cells. Application of normally sensitizing chemicals to skin devoid of Langerhans cells (skin treated with corticosteroids, UVB light, or cellophane adhesive tape) does not induce contact sensitivity and may produce specific immunologic tolerance to the contactant."[58]

"Coincident with the development of DTH during infection is a widespread activation of free and fixed mononuclear phagocytes throughout the body. Tissue macrophages develop profound alterations in morphology, cell proliferation, phagocytosis, and the capacity to destroy intracellular and extracellular microorganisms. Each of these changes is dependent on interactions with sensitized lymphocytes. These systemic changes in the antimicrobial activity of immunologically activated macrophages may explain observations made as early as 1936 that animals responding to reinfection with one microorganism (bacterium A) acquire the ability to resist nonspecifically infection with antigenically unrelated pathogens (bacterium B, C, or D). Unlike the long-lived, antigen specific, DTH response, this nonspecific element of acquired resistance is short lived and can only be reexpressed by further exposure to the original microbe (bacterium A) [*ed.* DNCB acts in the same way].

"Thus the DTH response to foreign antigens induces a series of immune reactions whose ultimate purpose is the short-term accumulation of nonspecifically cytotoxic, macrophage effector cells. Mononuclear phagocytes rapidly and preferentially accumulate at sites of infection. These inflammatory cells co-locate with antigen-reactive, sensitized T-cells and undergo dramatic changes in their functional state. The activated macrophages that result are pleuripotent cytotoxic effector cells which destroy viruses, bacteria, fungi, single and multicellular parasites, allografts, and tumor cells. This complex network of cell-mediated reactions is controlled by an even more complex interaction of various cytokines, those released by the T-cell, the macrophage, and even the target cell. DTH reactions are not self-destructive overreactions to foreign antigens, but rather tightly controlled body defenses against tissue allografts, infection, and neoplastic change."[59]

DNCB Treatment Instructions
(Rev. 12/1/93)
Billi Goldberg

DNCB is a potent topical contact sensitizer. Studies have shown that, when used regularly, DNCB will boost the immune response resulting in increased numbers of cytotoxic T-lymphocytes (CTL) and natural killer (NK) cells. Recent articles in *AIDS Treatment News* and *Treatment Update* provide additional information on DNCB that may be helpful.[60]

Drugs and Immunosuppression

Antibiotics, nucleosides analogues, and other drug treatments can interfere with the cell-mediated immune response and negate the systemic action initiated by DNCB. Drugs required for the treatment of infections must be continued until the infections are cleared or controlled. Prophylactic drugs can impair the immune response and might interfere with the immune boosting properties of DNCB. Individuals with AIDS must use PCP prophylaxis. The need, amount, and dosing schedule for other prophylactic drugs and treatments that suppress absolute CD8 counts should be given serious consideration. *It is extremely important to avoid all forms of ultraviolet radiation such as sunlight (wear a hat and use sunblock) and tanning salons. UV light not only suppresses cellular immunity but can increase HIV replication.*

Vitamins, Minerals, Herbs and Immunity

Individuals with compromised immune systems fighting chronic infections require supplements of basic vitamins and minerals. Suggested supplements are Multimineral tab, Multivitamin tab, Beta Carotene (25,000 I.U.), B-Complex, Vitamin C (1,000 mg.), Vitamin E (400 I.U.), Odorless Garlic (270 mg.), and Zinc (60 mg.). These supplements can be taken once or twice a day; however, Zinc should only be taken once a day since it can be toxic when over 100 mg. per day is used. There are studies that show that the optimal amount of Vitamin C is one to three grams per day with amounts over that causing interference with the immune response. NAC can also cause immunosuppression.

Most herbs are polysaccharides that initiate a systemic antibody response or Th2. Studies have shown that activation of this Th2 response will shutdown the cell-mediated immune response (Th1) required to control the infections involved in AIDS. Herbs, therefore, should not be used indiscriminately or on a regular basis unless it can be shown that they initiate cellular immunity or delayed-type hypersensitivity. Herbs should *not* be used unless the immunological action is known.

Initial Application*(if previous DNCB user, start with 0.2 percent Solution)*

1. Using a cotton swab, apply the **10 percent Solution** to the inner LEFT forearm in a 2x2-inch square. (Do not use with thymic peptides or cytokines.)

2. After a few minutes, apply the swab with the **10 percent Solution** a second time on the same 2x2-inch square location.

3. Let dry for a few minutes and cover with a large adhesive bandage, making certain that the adhesive does not touch the application site. Do not remove bandage or wash the application site for at least ten hours.

4. Do not, under any conditions, apply DNCB again until two weeks has elapsed, even if there is no reaction at the application site.

After Two Weeks

1. Using a swab, apply the **2 percent Solution** to the inner RIGHT forearm in a 2x2-inch square.

2. After a few minutes, apply the swab with the **2 percent Solution** a second time on the same 2x2-inch square location.

3. Let dry for a few minutes and cover with a large adhesive bandage, making certain that the adhesive does not touch the application site. Do not remove bandage or wash the application site for at least ten hours.

4. In less than seventy-two hours, the skin at the application site should be bright red, itchy, and slightly raised. If this happens, start weekly applications as per the next section.

5. If there is no reaction, continue with weekly applications of the **10 percent Solution** (alternating arms each week) until there is an appropriate response at the application site, then start weekly applications.

After One Week And Each Week Thereafter

1. Repeat steps 1–4 above, using the **2 percent Solution,** *and using a different application site for each weekly application.* Stinging at the site within one hour after application is a sign of an appropriate dose that will result in a good reaction, but this does not occur in all individuals.

2. It is advisable to move the application site each month between the inner arms, inner thighs, and trunk. It is especially important to apply DNCB on the upper and lower trunk areas more often that other sites, since the lungs and gastrointestinal tract are primary sources of opportunistic infections. Peyer's patches

(PP) are lymph nodes in the small intestine and must be activated. When applying to the trunk area, use a 3x3-inch square.
Every six weeks (more often if there are infections), it is advisable to use extra DNCB by applying the swab one additional
time to the trunk area application site.

3. If the application site is not bright red and slightly raised in
twenty-four to seventy-two hours, the solution is too weak. For
the next application, either increase the solution strength or
apply one extra application with the swab.

4. If the skin at the application site has raised blisters or open sores,
decrease the strength of the application by either applying only
once with the swab, or using a weaker solution, such as 0.2 percent or 0.02 percent.

5. If the present application site becomes bright red in twenty-four
to seventy-two hours or any previous application site changes
color, you are considered sensitized and need only to continue
applications on a weekly basis.

6. Do not use DNCB more than *once a week,* no matter what conditions or circumstances occur.

If severe contact dermatitis or itching occurs, apply calamine lotion,
aloe vera, cocoa butter, or a topical disinfectant such as Bactine
directly to the rash. The use of cortisone or hydrocortisone creams
is not recommended, as they have systemic immunosuppressing
effects. An overly strong reaction resulting in dermatitis is a sign of
an excellent immune response; this is a positive rather than a negative
sign. The dermatitis will heal in time and will not leave a scar.

*DNCB must be used weekly to be effective and to initiate appropriate
systemic immune responses.*

Supplemental DNCB Information
Billi Goldberg

The following information is to assist those who do not have access to
a readily available supply of DNCB (1-Chloro-2,4-dinitrobenzene
[$C_6H_3ClN_2O_4$]).

Manufacture

DNCB is produced in crystal form by a number of chemical companies in most countries. It can only be ordered for human use in the USA by authorized medical doctors or researchers. For industrial or business purposes, it can be obtained by the company representative using its resale number. For example, a company involved in color photography might order DNCB from Eastman Kodak Company. DNCB purity should be at least ninety-eight percent.

Containers

The appropriate containers for DNCB are amber-colored, 5 dram vials. Use only molded polyseal caps to prevent evaporation of the acetone. These polyseal caps do not come with the bottle and must be ordered separately. If these caps are not used the acetone can evaporate, resulting in a much stronger solution strength, the use of which can cause severe dermatitis. Each container should be clearly marked with appropriate solution strength.

Status

DNCB is not approved for manufacture as a drug or as a treatment for HIV/AIDS. It is occasionally applied as a topical treatment for refractory warts and alopecia areata (hair loss probably caused by autoimmunity). It has also been used successfully in humans as a treatment for malignant melanoma and as immunotherapy for skin lesions. DNCB can be used weekly after sensitization to check for cellular immunity (anergy). Approved methods of checking for anergy (PPD and Multitest) are not considered accurate in individuals who are immunosuppressed.

Usage

Due to possible deleterious reactions, DNCB *should not to be used* with any exogenous cytokine treatment such as interleukins, growth factors, thymic peptides, and interferons.

DNCB should only be applied topically (externally) using appropriate treatment instructions. *Never ingest DNCB, or take it internally.* If proper treatment instructions are followed, DNCB has not demonstrated toxicity at recommended application/dosage. Contact dermatitis can result if too much solution is used, or if it is applied at a greater than recommended frequency. Evaporation of the acetone will cause the percentage of DNCB in the solution to increase, resulting in severe blistering, reddening, and itching. To prevent evaporation, DNCB should be refrigerated if at all possible. If in doubt about the strength of old solution, discard it and replace with new solution.

Preparation

> **10 percent solution:** Dissolve 12 grams of DNCB crystals in ½ cup of acetone.
> **2 percent solution:** Dissolve 2.4 grams of DNCB crystals in ½ cup of acetone.
> **0.2 percent solution:** Dissolve 0.24 grams of DNCB crystals in ½ cup of acetone.
> **0.02 percent solution:** Dissolve 0.024 grams of DNCB crystals in ½ cup of acetone.

DNCB solution is best stored in small amber bottles, using special leak-proof caps, and should be refrigerated and replaced after six months.

Be careful when preparing the DNCB crystal-acetone solution. Use rubber gloves (over clear plastic gloves), and avoid contact with the solution. Use a large pipet and a pipet helper to fill bottles from the solution containers. A liquid handling bottle-top dispenser is also suitable for filling bottles, as is a dispenser with a petcock such as those used in large-volume wine containers. It is simplest to just pour the solution into each bottle. If DNCB solution spills on any exposed bodily surface, wash immediately with soap and water.

Mixing DNCB with lotions instead of acetone is not recommended, as this interferes with the absorption of the DNCB haptens by the skin.

DNCB/Acemannan Protocol for HIV/AIDS

Dinitrochlorobenzene (DNCB), a topical contact sensitizing agent, is the primary component of this therapy. Acemannan is used as a temporary adjuvant or enhancer of DNCB's effect for people whose immune systems have been too damaged to readily respond to DNCB. This protocol should only be used under the care of a licensed physician, or the guidance of some one with clinical familiarity with its use in HIV/AIDS.

1. The first step is to establish sensitization to DNCB according to treatment instructions. (In cases of profound illness, DNCB and Acemannan may be begun at the same time.)

2. Select the form and route of administration for the Acemannan component of the therapy. For asymptomatic seropositives, DNCB alone is sufficient as therapy, and Acemannan is not recommended. For those who are mildly to moderately symptomatic, or have moderately low absolute CD8 counts (less than 750), oral Acemannan is recommended. Individuals with clear AIDS-defining opportunistic infections, or dangerously low absolute CD8 counts (less than 400), should use low dose veterinary Acemannan immunostimulant intravenously.

DNCB with Oral Acemannan

The DeVeras Beverage contains 1,200 mg of Acemannan per liter. Add five or six drops of vinegar to the bottle upon opening and refrigerate the open product. Each dose should be consumed with food or milk in the stomach, even if only a small amount. Many people take a small amount (4–6 oz.) of whole milk or a spoonful of ice cream prior to each dose of the beverage.

For those who are moderately symptomatic with HIV disease, begin the protocol as follows, after sensitization with DNCB:

1. Beginning on Friday evening, consume two one-liter bottles of the aloe beverage over a thirty-six-hour period. Use small divided doses (about five ounces at a time over the course of Friday evening and Saturday). Complete the full two liters before retiring on Saturday.

2. On Sunday afternoon, apply the weekly application of DNCB (Follow DNCB Treatment Instructions, pp. 105–108).

3. If Acemannan capsules can be obtained from a Canadian source, twenty capsules (100 mg. each) should be consumed at intervals in the same manner over the course of thirty-six hours (Fri-

day evening/Saturday). DNCB is applied on Sunday afternoon, as outlined above.

4. Monitor your progress by following absolute CD8 counts and your subjective feeling of health improvement, energy level, appetite, weight gain, etc.

5. Upon complete resolution of all symptoms of disease, use oral Acemannan for an additional week, then discontinue. Continue with DNCB indefinitely.

6. Upon sensitization to DNCB, and after two weeks of Acemannan therapy, all prophylactic antibiotics, antifungals, and antivirals, except PCP prophylaxis, should be discontinued. Use oral Acemannan intermittently while continuing weekly applications of DNCB, should any disease symptoms appear.

DNCB with Injectable Acemannan

Acemannan Immunostimulant is approved for use only in veterinary medicine. However, you may be able to obtain it through the treatment underground or from a sympathetic veterinarian. Each vial contains 10 mg. of sterile injectable-grade drug. The IV protocol is only recommended for those with opportunistic disease and/or very low (less than 400) absolute CD8 counts. In cases of life-threatening illness, DNCB and IV Acemannan may be begun at the same time. For best results, DNCB sensitization should be achieved first if at all possible. For those suffering from severe HIV disease use the following protocol as a rescue or salvage therapy.

1. Acemannan Immunostimulant comes in a kit containing two vials—one containing the lyophilized drug and one containing a sterile saline diluent. First, wipe the sterile diluent bottle's rubber seal with alcohol. Then, using a 10 cc syringe and a 21 or 22 gauge needle, insert and draw up 10 cc of the clear fluid. Sterilize the vial containing Acemannan as above (wipe the rubber cap with alcohol), and then insert and evacuate the syringe containing the saline diluent. This reconstitutes the drug into its fluid form. Allow to sit for ten minutes and shake vigorously before using.

2. Avoid the use of aspirin, acetaminophen, or ibuprofen on the day of the treatment. Never insert a needle into the vial containing the reconstituted drug without first wiping the rubber

seal with alcohol and using a sterilized needle.

3. On Friday evening, using sterile technique, draw 1 cc of solution and inject intravenously. For ten minutes after the injection, observe yourself carefully for respiratory distress. If this occurs, immediately use a bronchodilator inhaler, such as Primatene Mist or Alupent.

4. During the first twenty-four to seventy-two hours after the injection, observe for fever, chills, muscle and joint aches, headache, and flu symptoms. These are a "desirable" effects, evidence of profound immune stimulation. If you develop these symptoms, reduce the weekly dose to ½ cc, and remain at that dose for the duration of Acemannan therapy. If no immune response is elicited, the dose may be increased to 2 ccs per week for no more than three weeks. The following week, reduce the dose to 1 cc for two weeks, and then to ½ cc for the remaining duration of Acemannan therapy. Eventually, everyone will develop at least mild symptoms indicative of immune stimulation from Acemannan. Higher doses are counterproductive due to the large amount of antibodies produced by this polysaccharide drug. If you are persistently nonresponsive, positive results may be achieved by increasing the size of the area on the skin to which DNCB is applied and using the maximum dosage that may be tolerated without severe burn. (This may entail increasing the DNCB dose to three swabs of the your usual dose, and increasing the size of the area of skin treated to 4x4-inch square on the trunk.)

After it has been determined that you are responding to IV Acemannan, 400 mg. of ibuprofen (Motrin, Advil) may be taken two hours prior to treatment, and then every six hours as needed to allay drug-related discomfort.

After one month of therapy, all prophylactic drugs (except for PCP prophylaxis) should be stopped or curtailed, or the protocol simply won't work. As symptoms abate, general health improves to a satisfactory level, and CD8s remain consistently higher than 750, discontinue Acemannan completely and continue with weekly DNCB indefinitely. Should symptoms emerge and recur, use the DeVeras beverage or Acemannan capsules per protocol for a brief period.

Improvement warranting discontinuation of IV Acemannan is

generally anticipated within six months (maximum) of initiating therapy. *Most people will only require between four to twelve weekly treatments.* Particular attention should be made to proper nutrition, including appropriate supplements. Antioxidant supplements, such as Twinlabs brand "Oxy-quenchers," and a multivitamin and multimineral combination tablet, are recommended. Avoid Chinese herbs entirely while on this protocol. Further research on their composition is needed before their use in combination with other therapies can be evaluated.

If you must use antibiotic drugs as treatment for limited periods of time, it is advisable to use ½ cc of Acemannan injected once or twice a month to help offset the immunosuppressive properties of these antibiotic drugs.

This protocol is not "written in stone," but the parameters and limitations outlined here are based on clinical observation of hundreds of patients who have achieved a degree of immunorestoration. It is imperative that Acemannan be discontinued when warranted by the above criteria. Lifelong maintenance therapy with DNCB is the desired goal. Practitioners or patients skilled in using the protocol may develop some variances in the treatment regimen. However, I must caution, that after seven years of studying the pharmacokinetics of Acemannan, I have concluded that higher doses pose serious clinical problems, a discussion of which is beyond the scope of this essay.

In nonresponsive patients, a brief elevation of Acemannan to 2 cc per week, followed by a dramatic drop in dosage, first by half, and then by half again (to ½ cc) over the course of a few weeks, achieves the desired fever and aches. The reason for this is not clearly understood at this time. Based on extensive personal clinical experience, and comparing notes with clinicians using variations on the protocol, the key to this therapy rests in the ability to skillfully discern the lowest possible dose of Acemannan that will be effective. More important, it is vital to understand when to stop Acemannan therapy and proceed only with weekly treatment of DNCB.

For the rationale behind this treatment protocol, please see Acemannan *(pages 74–77),* Macrophage Activation by Direct Stimulation *(pages 98–102), and* How DNCB Works *(pages 102–105).*

Alternative Treatments for Herpes, Cytomegalovirus and Varicella Zoster Infections

In the absence of a competent immune system, lipid-coated viruses have greater opportunity to invade and damage the host system. Viruses, unlike other pathogenic microorganisms, are known as obligate intracellular parasites. A virus invades the host cell, and takes over particles of the DNA strands at the center of the cell, altering the cell's genetic machinery so that it produces viral proteins by which it produces "copies" of itself. This continues until the cell's resources are used up, at which time the cell ruptures, spilling its viral copies into the bloodstream where they travel to infect new cells.

A certain class of viruses, known as lipid-coated viruses, use a fatty coating made of substances from within the host system. The viral proteins that would otherwise be recognized as foreign and destroyed by the immune system elude this defense by surrounding their genetic material with proteins and fats made from substances in the body not recognized as foreign, making their presence difficult for the immune system to detect.

Lipid-coated viruses include Herpes Simplex Viruses 1 and 2 (HSV-1, HSV-2), Varicella-Zoster Virus(VZV)—the cause of shingles, Epstein-Barr virus (EBV) which has been implicated in causing Chronic Fatigue Immune Dysfunction Syndrome (CFIDS), and Cytomegalovirus (CMV), a major cause of blindness and death among people with AIDS. These viruses escape immune system detection by "hiding out" in various cells such as B-lymphocytes, monocytes/macrophages, and neurons (nerve clusters), where they can remain dormant for long periods of time. They can be activated by stress, diet changes, illness, or sudden decline in immune status.

Conventional medicine has been very unsuccessful in treating viruses in general, and lipid-coated viruses in particular. Widely used drugs for the treatment of these virus are toxic, expensive, and, in many cases, relatively ineffective.

This fact sheet will outline some natural and affordable treatment choices that you may include in your total health maintenance program. These can serve both as treatments for syndromes associated with these viruses, as well as preventing symptomatic activation of latent viral infections.

BHT

Butylated Hydroxytuolene is a food preservative widely used to prevent rancidity in fat-containing foods. It is believed to strip lipid-coated viruses of their protective envelope, leaving the virus susceptible to recognition and destruction by the immune system. It is also thought to remove the binding proteins that viruses use to penetrate cell membranes.

BHT is widely available at buyer's clubs and health food retailers, both in capsules and powdered form. Researchers believe that 250 mg. taken daily with a fat containing meal will prevent outbreaks of herpes, and 500 mg. daily during acute outbreaks will shorten the length and decrease the severity of the outbreak.[61] In the case of shingles, higher dosages may be needed.

It is thought that 2,000 to 3,000 mg. of BHT will stop the progressions of symptoms of CMV disease, and that after a period of treatment for acute symptoms, the dosage can be decreased to 1,000 mg. per day to prevent reactivation. Chronic Fatigue Immune Dysfunction Syndrome associated with the Epstein-Barr virus has been reported to abate when treated with BHT at a 1,000 mg. daily dose. The substance is metabolized with fats in the system, thus ingesting it with fatty foods is suggested. In the case of acute, serious viral illnesses, such as shingles, CMV, or disseminated herpes, it is suggested that the measured dose of powder be mixed with olive oil and allowed to sit overnight prior to consuming.

Hypericin

This chemical is an extract from the St. John's Wort plant, traditionally known to farmers as goatweed. It has a long history of use in Europe as an antidepressant medication.

Hypericin should only be used as an alternative treatment for a specific condition and not on a regular basis for prophylaxis or as an HIV retroviral treatment. Not only does it result in a photosensitive condition which suppresses the cellular immune response and interferes with delayed-type hypersensitivity, but it is believed to activate the antibody system. The increased activation of antibodies has been shown to suppress cellular immunity and, possibly, result in B-cell lymphomas.

Researchers now believe that at least 10 mg. per day of pure hypericin are necessary for inactivating lipid viruses. Experiments with mice, traditionally seen as a good model for human immune research, have shown herpes and cytomegalovirus to be readily inactivated in a minimum of time, using the correct concentrations of hypericin.

Persons using hypericin may develop photosensitivity, and should thus avoid unnecessary exposure to sunlight. In theory, it is possible that hypericin may be used to inactivate herpes, CMV, and EBV infections. When symptoms abate, hypericin may be gradually phased out over a period of time, and replaced with a gradually increasing dose of BHT, which is much more affordable and easier to obtain. *See Resource Guide, page 154.*

Chinese Herbs

Western university research has in the last few years demonstrated clear antiviral activity of commonly used traditional Chinese medicinal herbs. Many have been shown to be extremely effective against Epstein-Barr, herpes, and cytomegalovirus. Western laboratory research has shown them to have immunomodulatory properties, in addition to their antiviral properties.

Misha Cohen, O.M.D., founder of the Quan Yin Clinic, has developed a patented formula of dried herbal extracts as an adjunctive therapy for acute cytomegalovirus infection. Cohen reports an enhancement of the effect of standard treatments as well as some amelioration of the side effects of gancyclovir and foscanet by the addition of the herbal formula to the therapeutic regime. It is known that Chinese medicinal herbs are useful in treating specific disorders; however, it appears that daily prophylactic consumption of polysaccharide herbs can contribute to antibody production, and would therefore presumably be contraindicated as anti-HIV therapy. *See Resource Guide, page 153.*

Membrane Fluidizers

Prior to the advent of reverse transcriptase-inhibiting drugs, many people used nutritional substances made from egg and soy lecithin, due to some promising antiviral research done at the Weizmann Institute in Rehovat, Israel. It was theorized that the cholesterol in the external membranes of T-cells and in the lipid coatings of viruses produced structural rigidity essential for binding of virus to the target host cell. These so-called membrane fluidizers are believed to extract cholesterol from the cell walls of viral lipid coat and the cell membranes of T-cells, causing a fluidity of interaction between virus and host, and reducing infectivity.

Many people reported some degree of success using these products as a treatment for HIV. The limited formal research done in human medicine for HIV treatment was not very promising. Yet there were reported cases of arrested viral disease progression for people suffering from hepatitis and CMV. A number of therapeutic benefits have been ascribed to the use of nontoxic lecithin extracts. Many people have reported receiving some relief from the gastrointestinal problems associated with CMV, and some have anecdotally reported the cessation of clinical decline, including vision loss and other symptoms associated with CMV disease.

When the product was in more widespread use, people were generally using up from ten to thirty grams per day, driving the product cost from thirty dollars to ninety dollars per month. A home formula made from a soy lecithin extract may be made using Twinlabs brand PC-55. This form of the treatment can cost as low as fifty cents per day to use. *See Resource Guide, page 154.*

Monolaurin

This nutritional product is believed to have a mode of action similar to that of the lecithin extracts. It is a saturated fatty acid, a chemical constituent of mother's milk (known to confer immunity on nursing infants until the evolution of independent immunity). It is known to be safe, and is licensed by the USDA as a food additive for the purpose of preventing the growth of bacteria and viruses in food products. It has demonstrated antiviral activity against lipid viruses. It is available in most health food stores at a cost of about thirty dollars per month. Many people use this substance in combination with BHT as a CMV prophylaxis.

Dietary Interventions

There are some nutritional interventions which may help prevent the development of CMV and other herpes virus symptoms. Viruses in this family have a lipid coat rich in arginine, an amino acid. To make its protective coating, the virus must use excess arginine from the host system provided by foods rich in this amino acid, including almonds, barley, beer, chocolate, fresh corn, and many types of nuts. The amino acid lysine's chemical makeup most closely resembles arginine. In the absence of arginine, the virus will attempt to use lysine in the construction of its protective coating; however, with lysine, the virus is not able to complete this process and is destroyed. An increase in intake of lysine, a very affordable nutritional supplement, along with a decrease in dietary intake of arginine-rich foods, is believed to help keep herpes and CMV infections dormant and harmless. Lysine is available in most health food stores and is generally assumed to be safe.

Based on research on nutrition and unconventional medical technologies, it is clear that there are always measures that can be taken to avoid a seemingly unavoidable medical disaster. Those who face the challenge and seek out solutions from wherever they may be found are the most likely to achieve the most positive results. For those willing to cast aside preconceptions, keep an open mind, do their homework, and muster up the courage to do what feels right for them, there is hope. It is a very personal choice.

Chinese Herbs for HIV: A Critical Analysis
Charles R. Caulfield and Billi Goldberg

Important and seminal Western-style university research has been published on the biological activity of herbs used routinely in the treatment of HIV by practitioners of Traditional Chinese Medicine (TCM). The immune modulating properties of these agents have

been shown to fall into various and distinct categories of immunological activity.

In "Immunomodulating Chinese Herbal Medicines," author Li
Xiao-Yu of the Shanghai Institute of Materia Medica, Chinese Academy of Sciences, outlines the immune activities of six natural herbal
products, based on recent research on the immunotoxicology of Chinese medicinal herbs. These herbs are clearly active immunologically,
and can modulate, potentiate, or suppress the immune response.[62]

Surprisingly, the most popular of these herbs have been shown
to induce antibody production, which, based on current knowledge,
would presumably be contraindicated in HIV/AIDS. Western medical
immunology has made available a new analysis and understanding of
Chinese therapeutics. Understanding this new theory, and its relevance to treating HIV/AIDS, has become indispensable to clinicians
from all disciplines. Chinese medicine can only hope to function in full
partnership with Western medicine if it heeds the most recent discoveries in immunology.

In recent months, the medical and lay press have widely discussed
the purpose and cross-inhibitory roles of the Th1 and Th2 immune
cascades.[63] Th1, or cell-mediated immunity, operates through the
process of delayed-type hypersensitivity, utilizing cytotoxic T-lymphocytes and natural killer cells as its antimicrobial strategy. It provides defense against infective organisms which actually enter the
cell and exist there as parasites.[64] Therefore, cellular immunity must
be upregulated to become the predominant immune response in
order to control the intracellular infections and HIV viral burden.[65]

The clinical evidence of induced cellular immunity, based on the
most current scientific research, would include elevations in numbers and activation of cytotoxic T-lymphocytes and natural killer cells.
These are now known to be the antimicrobial mechanisms of this
cascade.[66]

Therapeutic use of polysaccharides (complex carbohydrates), the
physiologically active components of many Chinese herbs, are now
described in standard 1993 textbook science as falling into the general
classification of T-cell independent antigens (T-ind). These are capable of activating B-cells, and therefore antibodies, without the facili-
tation of T-cell help.

According to the standard text *Immunology,* many polysaccharides fall into this category. The text states, "in particular, they [polysaccharides] are all large polymeric molecules with repeating antigenic determinants Many possess the ability, at high concentrations, to activate B-cell clones that are specific for other antigens (polyclonal B-cell activation) [mainly T-cell independent antigens]...."[67] These antigens are particularly resistant to degradation. This implies that polyclonal activating polysaccharides remain in the metabolic pool for long periods of time, due to their durable chemical linkage, initiating a protracted, nonspecific, long-term induction of humoral response. Based of factual scientific knowledge, about 30 percent of ocurrences of AIDS-related lymphomas have been attributed to polyclonal stimulation of B-cells.[68] There is also the distinct possibility that antibodies and complement to HIV, formed as a result of the nonspecific humoral response, may result in enhancement of infection in susceptible cells such as macrophages.[69]

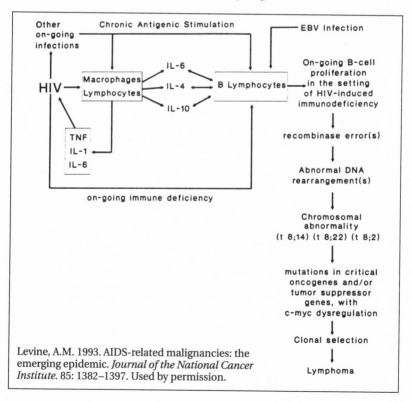

Levine, A.M. 1993. AIDS-related malignancies: the emerging epidemic. *Journal of the National Cancer Institute.* 85: 1382–1397. Used by permission.

Outlined below is a brief and preliminary review of the immune modulating activities of some commonly used herbs. It is important to note that the effects seen with herb usage may not be due to the purified version or extracts of the herb, but the entire composition of the plant, including other unknown and unrecognized substances.

Astragalus Mongholicus

Oddly enough, according to the paper by Li, some of the most commonly-used herbs in the treatment of HIV have profiles which classify them as Th2, thus B-cell activating. This property could rationally be expected to impair the cellular immune response. Astragalus is a principal example of this phenomenon. In spite of the almost universal use of this herb in TCM's treatment of HIV/AIDS, and the knowledge of its immune stimulating activities, its biological activity is largely confined to the humoral cascade, which, as we have shown, is potentially harmful in the long run for people with HIV.[70] According to Li, "this [astragalus] herb polysaccharide enlarges the spleen *and increases antibody formation.* While it promoted significantly mice macrophage phagocytosis, it only marginally effects lymphocyte proliferation."

Acanthopanax Senticosus and Eleutheroccocus Senticosus

The root of these plants is commonly used as a tonic, an adaptogen, and a sedative agent. They occur in numerous HIV tonic formulations. Despite the fact that Dr. Li describes this herb as possessing "significant immunopotentiating action," its principal mode of action is in its ability to "potentiate the antibody response." Another herb in the same family, Acanthopanax gracilistylus, is also known as an "adaptogen." It has been shown to be "biologically active by its containing a triterpine compound which increases antibody formation and T-lymphocyte proliferation." In light of current knowledge, it is safe to surmise, that B-cell induced antibody production precipitated increases in CD4 T-lymphocytes of the Th2 lineage which then serve in the capacity of "antibody helper cells." Beyond conjecture, this proves that Acanthopanax, and its aforementioned herbal cousins, induce a counterproductive Th2 response, thereby impairing the critical cell-mediated or Th1 response.

Panax Notoginseng

Other commonly used herbs in the PWA community have pharmacological profiles making it difficult to assess the type of immune cascade elicited. Prominent among these is Panax, a famous traditional herb grown in Southwest China having multiple modes of action. According to Dr. Li, this herb functions as an analgesic, tonic, and hematostatic, all presumably useful actions in HIV treatment. However, it has been determined that the combined saponin profile of this herb causes a marked increase in serum complement, a humoral immune mechanism, along with the promotion of antibodies. According to H.W. Yeung, et al., the saponins can selectively suppress delayed-type hypersensitivity which "may be related to their steroid-like structure."[71]

Aconitum

Alkaloids extracted from three different species of this herb were shown to be active as analgesics, antiinflammatory and immunosuppressive. While these properties are eminently useful in the management of autoimmune disease and inflammatory processes, they appear to do so by impairment of splenic activity (Western anatomical spleen vs. TCM spleen). Its mode of action has been compared to corticosteroids such as prednisone, and have little discernible application to HIV disease. It is known that activation of the complement component of the humoral system, will increase antibody production, inhibit vascular permeability, and impair leukocyte migratory responses.

Dr. Li's research at the Shanghai Academy of Sciences has identified two herbs, Artemisiae annua and Tripterigium wilfordii, not commonly used in HIV herbal formulations, which may be promising as inducers of the cellular immune response, and suppression of polyclonal antibody production depending on the specific active ingredients that are utilized. In addition to these, the indigenous American herb, Echinacea purpurea, may have value for use in immunocompromised individuals. But much more study is required, including in vivo testing along with regular evaluation of clinical parameters. It appears that no polysaccharides should be taken on a daily or regular basis because of their tendency to cause polyclonal anti-body formation and, therefore, suppression of cellular immunity. As with all pharmacologically active plant derivatives, the risk of developing tolerance must also be considered—possibly warranting rotation of cellular immunity facilitating herbs.

Artemisiae annua

This herb, frequently used as an adjunctive to basic HIV herbal formulations, has been used as an antimalarial treatment for thousands of years. The pure extract, artimisinine (Qing-haosu) is known to possess potent and rapid efficacy on malaria, particularly fulminating and cerebral malaria, which is notoriously difficult to treat. Although the evidence for the presumed effect of this herb is circumstantial, it is critical to note that in one study with symptomatic malaria infected mice, easily achievable blood levels of this herb lowered serum circulating immune-complexes (evidence of artemisia's ability to downregulate the humoral response). At least superficially, it appears to effectively enhance the cell-mediated immune response to a significant extent. According to Dr. Li, "Artemether, [artemsia derivative] ... lowered circulating serum immune-complexes, maintained normal red blood counts ... and protected the infected mice from death." Since immune-complexes of HIV are considered to be an integral part of lymph node destruction in the pathogenesis of AIDS, perhaps there is a role for artemether in lowering the circulating HIV immune-complexes.[72] In a study by Tawfix, et al., three derivatives—artemisinin, dihydroartemisinin, and arteether—showed a marked suppression of humoral responses but did not alter the delayed-type hypersensitivity response to sheep erythrocytes at the same dose levels. None of the three agents possessed any antiinflammatory activity, therefore they may have a selective immunosuppressive activity.[73]

Tripterigium wilfordii

This plant belongs to the phylum Celastraceae, and has undergone a sort of renaissance in China during the last twenty years, based on the observation of its effectiveness in treating rheumatoid arthritis, chronic nephritis, and chronic skin disorders, including lupus and psoriasis, all chronic immune disorders. The active chemicals are thought to be triptolide, tripdiolode, tripterine, euonine, and wilfor-trine. The extracts have been shown in convincing studies to have a potent antileukemia activity, and are documented to clearly have a pronounced immunosuppressant effect. Concomitant tumor-immunity was recorded. The negative side to this herb is that two of its active ingredients, tripterine and euonine, have been shown in mice studies to depress the delayed hypersensitivity reaction to dinitrochlorobenzene (DNCB).[74] The other active ingredients appeared to be depressant only on the humoral or antibody response, which could result in usefulness in the treatment of inflammatory or autoimmune diseases and might have some value in HIV/AIDS.

Echinacea purpurea

There is little question that this herb is a pure and potent polysaccharide, able to initiate T-cell independent antibody responses. Macrophages appear to be the main target of echinacea, resulting in their activation and resultant secretion of Tumor Necrosing Factor-alpha, Interleukins 1 and 6, and the induction of macrophage production of reactive oxygen intermediates, free radicals which are a primary method of macrophage therapeutic cytotoxicity.[75] Echinacea also appears to stimulate bone marrow production of polymorphonuclear granulocytes.[76] According to S.S. Hendler, M.D., Ph.D. in *The Doctors' Vitamin and Mineral Encyclopedia,* "There is some contradictory, but unconfirmed, evidence suggesting that echinacea might actually depress T4 helper cell activity in *some* people. Anyone who is immune deficient should use echinacea only while being monitored by a physician so that the effect of the herb on the immune system can be reliably evaluated."[77] Conventional wisdom may contraindicate the long-term use of this herb due to possible toxicity associated with stimulation of the lipopolysaccharide receptor in macrophages.

It would seem reckless for Chinese medicine to disregard the recent developments in immunology merely because they seem to contradict long and dearly held notions. A new study shows that mucosa-associated lymphoid tissue (MALT) immune responses, involving the gastrointestinal tract (GI), and initiated by IgA anti-protein antibodies, are Th2 cell dependent.[78] Ginseng, a well-known traditional herb and polysaccharide, induces a significant increase of serum corticosterone along with the production of antibodies, both of which suppress cellular immunity.[79] The fact remains that diagnostic technology now exists by which Chinese medicine may revise and improve its approach to treating AIDS, as well as to use the Western diagnostics as clear demonstration of the efficacy of certain herbal treatment strategies. Ultimately, this will further its goal to function as a viable complementary and adjunctive set of strategies in concert with Western allopathic medicine.

It should also be noted that these considerations are of paramount importance singularly in AIDS. This appears to be possibly the only disease in which a counterproductive immunological cascade (Th2) acquires a competitive advantage, thereby impairing the natural ebb and flow between cellular and humoral immunity. In healthy individuals, these essentially function as complementary cascades. In the case of HIV disease and, possibly, Chronic Fatigue Immune Dysfunction Syndrome (CFIDS), however, the deleterious Th2 response acquires disproportionate predominance, inhibiting its Th1 counterpart, which is the key to managing AIDS-related illness.

Notes

Antioxidant Therapies for HIV

1. Pearson, D., Shaw, S. 1980. *Life Extension.* New York: Warren Books.
2. O'Connor, T., Gonzalez-Nunez, A. 1987. *Living with AIDS: Reaching Out.* San Francisco: Corwin Publishers.

Acemannan

3. Yates, K. M., Rosenberg, L. J., Harris, C. K., et al. 1992. Pilot study of the effect of acemannan in cats infected with feline immunodeficiency virus. *Veterinary Immunology and Immunopathology* 35:177–189.
4. Kahlon, J. B., Kemp, M.C., Yawei, N., et al. 1991. Inhibition of AIDS virus replication in vitro. *Molecular Biotherapy* 3:127–135.
5. Womble, D., Helderman, H. 1988. Enhancement of allo-responsiveness of human lymphocytes by acemannan (Carrisyn®). *International Journal of Immunopharmacology* 10:967–974.

Delayed Hypersensitivity Thearpy for HIV: DNCB

6. Mills, L. B. 1986. Stimulation of T-cellular immunity by cutaneous application of dinitrochlorobenzene. *Journal of the American Academy of Dermatology* 14:1089–1090.
7. Stricker, R. B., Elswood, B. F., Abrams, D. I. 1991. Dendritic cells and dinitrochlorobenzene (DNCB): a new treatment approach to AIDS. *Immunology Letters* 29:191–196.
8. Stricker, R. B., Zhu, Y. S., Gong, Y., et al. 1992. Pilot study of topical dinitrochlorobenzene (DNCB) in HIV disease: clinical features and molecular correlates. Amsterdam: *Proceedings of the Eighth International Conference on AIDS* PO-B3461 [abstract].
9. See: Hill, S., Edwards, A. J., Kimber, I., Knight, S. C. 1990. Systemic migration of dendritic cells during contact sensitization. *Immunology* 71:277–281; and Cumberbatch, M. and Kimber, I. 1992. Dermal tumour necrosis factor-α induces dendritic cell migration to

draining lymph nodes, and possibly provides one stimulus for Langerhans' cell migration. *Immunology* 75:257–263.

10. See: Macatonia, S. E., Taylor, P. M., Knight, S. C., Askonas, B. A. 1989. Primary stimulation by dendritic cells induces antiviral proliferative and cytotoxic T-cell responses in vitro. *Journal of Experimental Medicine* 169:1255–1264; and Macatonia, S. E., Patterson, S., Knight, S. C. Primary proliferative and cytotoxic T-cell responses to HIV induced in vitro. *Immunology* 74:399–506.

11. Meltzer, M. S., Nacy, C. A. 1989. Delayed type hypersensitivity and the induction of activated, cytotoxic macrophages. In: Paul, W. E., ed. 1989. *Fundamental Immunology,* Second Edition. New York: Raven Press, pp. 765–777.

12. See: Ullrich, R., Zeitz, M., Riecken, E. O. 1992. Enteric immunologic abnormalities in human immunodeficiency virus infection. *Seminars in Liver Disease* 12:167–174.

Natural Therapies for Candidiasis Infections

13. Block, E. 1985. The chemistry of garlic and onion. *Scientific American* 252:114–119.

Immune Modulating Nutrients: Vitamin A and Zinc

14. Information from: Marcus, R., Coulston, A. M. 1990. Fat-soluble vitamins. In: Gilman, A. G., Rall, T. W., Nies, A. S., Taylor, P., eds. 1990. *The Pharmacological Basis of Therapeutics,* New York: Pergamon Press, pp. 1553–1563; and Roitt, I. M., Delves, P. J., eds. 1992. *Encyclopedia of Immunology.* San Diego: Academic Press, pp. 1562–1563, 1577–1578.

Germanium: Potent Immune Modulator from Japan

15. Goodman, S. 1988. Therapeutic effects of organic germanium. *Medical Hypotheses* 207–215.

16. Sato. I., Yuan, B. D., Nishimura, T., Tanaka, N. 1985. Inhibition of tumor growth and metastasis in association with modification of immune response by novel organic germanium compounds. *Journal of Biological Response Modifiers* 4:159–168.

17. Aso, H., Suzuki, F., Yamaguchi, T., et al. 1985. Induction of interferon and activation of NK cells and macrophages in mice by oral

administration of Ge-132, an organic germanium compound. *Micro-biology and Immunology* 65–74.

18. Kobayashi, H., Aso, H., Ishida, N., et al. 1992. Preventive effect of a synthetic immunomodulator, 2-carboxyethylgermanium sesquioxide, on the generation of suppressor macrophages in mice immunized with allogeneic lymphocytes. *Immunopharmacology and Immunotoxicology* 14:841–64.

Vitamin C and Immunity

19. Muggli, R. 1992. Vitamin C and the immune system. In: Roitt, I. M., ed. 1992. *Encyclopedia of Immunology.* San Diego, CA: Academic Press, Inc.

20. See: Munster, A. M., Loadholdt, C. B., Leary, A. G., Barnes, M. A. 1977. The effect of antibiotics on cell- mediated immunity. *Surgery* 81:692–695; Anderson, R., Oosthuizen, R., Maritz, R., et al. 1980. The effects of increasing weekly doses of ascorbate on certain cellular and humoral immune functions in normal volunteers. *American Journal of Clinical Nutrition* 33:71–76; and Ramirez, I., Richie, E., Wang, Y. M., van Eys, J. 1980. Effect of ascorbic acid in vitro on lymphocyte reactivity to mitogens. *Journal of Nutrition* 110:2207–2215.

Chinese Medicine and HIV Disease

21. Li, X. Y. 1991. Immunomodulating Chinese Herbal Medicines. *Memorias do Instituto Oswaldo Cruz* 86(SII):159–164.

Cellular and Antibody Immune Responses in AIDS

22. See: Kaufmann, S. H. E. 1988. CD8+ T-lymphocytes in intracellular microbial infections. *Immunology Today* 9:168–174; Kaufmann, S. H. E. 1993. Immunity to intracellular bacteria. *Annual Review of Immunology* 11:129–165; Mody, C. H., Chen, G. H., Jackson, C., et al. 1993. Depletion of murine CD8+ T-cells in vivo decreases pulmonary clearance of a moderately virulent strain of *Cryptococcus neoformans. Journal of Laboratory and Clinical Medicine* 121:765–773; Dannenberg, A. M. 1991. Delayed-type hypersensitivity and cell-mediated immunity in the pathogenesis of tuberculosis. *Immunology Today* 12:228–233; and Flynn, J. L., Goldstein, M. M., Triebold, K. J., Koller, B., Bloom, B. R. 1992. Major histocompatibility complex class I-restricted

T-cells are required for resistance to *Mycobacterium tuberculosis infection. Proceedings of the National Academy of Sciences* 89:12013–12017.

23. Walker, B. D., Plata, F. 1990. Cytotoxic T-lymphocytes against HIV. *AIDS* 4:177–184.

24. Meltzer, M. S., Nacy, C. A. 1989. Delayed type hypersensitivity and the induction of activated, cytotoxic macrophages. In: Paul, W. E., ed. 1989. *Fundamental Immunology,* Second Edition. New York: Raven Press, pp. 765–777.

25. See: Romagnani, S. 1992. Human Th1 and Th2 subsets: regulation of differentiation and role in protection and immunopathology. *International Archives of Allergy and Immunology* 98:279–285; Sher, A., Gazzinelli, T., Oswald, I. P., Clerici, M., et al.1992. Role of T-cell derived cytokines in the downregulation of immune responses in parasitic and retroviral infection. *Immunological Reviews* 127:183–204; and Bloom, B. R., Salgame, P., Diamond, B. 1992. Revisiting and revising suppressor T-cells. *Immunology Today* 13:131–135.

26. See: Mosmann, T. R., Coffman, R. L. 1989. Heterogeneity of cytokine secretion patterns and functions of helper T-cells. *Advances in Immunology* 46:111–147; and Salgame P., Abrams J. S., Clayberger C., et al. 1991. Differing lymphokine profiles of functional subsets of human CD4 and CD8 T-cell clones. *Science* 254:279–282.

27. A example of this interplay of Th1/Th2 is discussed brilliantly in: Fitzgerald T.J. 1992. The Th1/Th2-like switch in syphilitic infection: is it detrimental? *Infection and Immunity* 60:3475–3479.

28. See: Clerici, M., Shearer, G. M. 1993. A Th1→Th2 switch is a critical step in the etiology of HIV infection. *Immunology Today* 14:107–111; and Ezzell, C. 1993. AIDS' unlucky strike: when T-cells would rather switch than fight. *Journal of NIH Research* 5:59–64.

29. Shearer, G. M., Clerici, M. 1992. T-helper cell immune dysfunction in asymptomatic, HIV-1-seropositive individuals: the role of Th1-Th2 cross-regulation. *Chemical Immunology* 54:21–43.

30. Lanzavecchia, A. 1993. Identifying strategies for immune intervention. *Science* 260:937–944.

31. See: Cohen, J. 1993. T-cell shift: key to AIDS therapy? *Science* 262:175–176; and Kanagawa, O., Vaupel, B. A., Gayama, S., et al. 1993. Resistance of mice deficient in IL-4 to retrovirus-induced immunodeficiency syndrome (MAIDS). Ibid:240–242.

End Game, or How HIV Causes AIDS

32. See: Giannetti, A., Zambruno, G., Cimarelli, A., et al. 1993. Direct detection of HIV-1 RNA in epidermal Langerhans cells of HIV-infected patients. *Journal of AIDS* 6:329–333; and Langhoff, E., Haseltine, W. A. 1992. Infection of accessory dendritic cells by human immunodeficiency virus type 1. *Journal of Investigative Dermatology* 99:89S–94S.

33. Mactonia, S. E., Patterson, S., Knight, S. C. 1989. Suppression of immune responses by dendritic cells infected with HIV. *Immunology* 67:285–289.

34. Janeway, C. A. 1992. The case of the missing CD4s. *Current Opinions in Biology* 2:359–361.

35. Knight, S. C., Stagg, A. J. 1993. Antigen-presenting cell types. *Current Opinion in Immunology* 5:374–382.

36. See: Steinman, R. 1991. The dendritic cell system and its role in immunogenicity. *Annual Review of Immunology* 9:271–296; and Knight, S. C., Stagg, A., Hill, S., et al. 1992. Development and function of dendritic cells in health and disease. *Journal of Investigative Dermatology* 99:33S–38S.

37. Knight, S. C., Macatonia, S. E., Patterson, S. 1993. Infection of dendritic cells with HIV1: virus load regulates stimulation and suppression of T-cell activity. *Research in Virology* 144:75–80.

38. Johnson, J. G., Jenkins, M. K. 1992. Co-stimulatory function of antigen-presenting cells. *Journal of Investigative Dermatology* 99:62S–65S.

39. See: Kaufmann, S. H. E. 1988. CD8+ T-lymphocytes in intracellular microbial infections. *Immunology Today* 9:168–174; and Kaufmann, S. H. E. 1993. Immunity to intracellular bacteria. *Annual Review of Immunology* 11:129–165.

40. See: Pantaleo, G., De Maria, A., Koenig, S., Butini, L., Moss, B., Baseler, M., Lane, H. C., Fauci, A. S. 1990. CD8+ T-lymphocytes of patients with AIDS maintain normal broad cytolytic function despite the loss of human immunodeficiency virus-specific cytotoxicity. *Proceedings of the National Academy of Sciences* 87:4818–4822; and Go, C., Lancki, D. W., Fitch, F. W., Miller, J. 1993. Anergized T-cell clones retain their cytolytic ability. *Journal of Immunology* 150:367–376.

41. Mactonia, S. E., Lau, R., Patterson, S., Pinching, A. J., Knight, S. C.

1990. Dendritic cell infection, depletion and dysfunction in HIV-infected individuals. *Immunology* 71:38–45.

42. Charmichael, A., Jin, X., Sissons, P., Borysiewicz, L. 1993. Quantitative analysis of the human immunodeficiency virus type 1 (HIV-1)-specific cytotoxic T-lymphocyte (CTL) response at different stages of HIV-1 infection: differential CTL responses to HIV-1 and Epstein-Barr Virus in Late Disease. *Journal of Experimental Medicine* 177:249–256.

43. Pantaleo, G., Koenig, S., Baseler, M., Lane, H. C., Fauci, A. S. 1990. Defective clonogenic potential of CD8+ T-lymphocytes in patients with AIDS. *Journal of Immunology* 144:1696–1704.

44. Helbert, M. R., L'age-Stehr, J., Mitchison, N. A. 1993. Antigen presentation, loss of immunological memory and AIDS. *Immunology Today* 14:340–343.

45. Meyaard, L., Schuitemaker, H., Miedema. F. 1993. T-cell dysfunction in HIV infection: anergy due to defective antigen-presenting cell function? *Immunology Today* 14:161–164.

46. Gardner, M. B. 1992. State of the art: AIDS vaccine development. *AmFAR AIDS/HIV Treatment* Directory 30 September, pp. 5–10.

Macrophage Activation by Direct Stimulation

47. See: Womble, D., Helderman, J. H. 1992. The impact of acemannan on the generation and function of cytotoxic T-lymphocytes. 1992. *Immunopharmacology and Immunotoxicology* 14(1&2):63–77; and Marshall, G. D. and Druck, J. P. 1993. In vitro stimulation of NK activity by acemannan (ACM). *Journal of Immunology* 150:241A #1381 [abstract].

48. See: Yates, K. M., Rosenberg, L. J., Harris, C. K., et al. 1992. Pilot study of the effect of acemannan in cats infected with feline immunodeficiency virus. *Veterinary Immunology and Immunopathology* 35:177–189; and Sheets, M. A., Unger, B. A., Giggleman, G. F., Tizard, I. R. 1991. Studies of the effect of acemannan on retrovirus infections: clinical stabilization of feline leukemia virus-infected cats. *Molecular Biotherapy* 3:41–45.

49. Meltzer, M. S., Gendelman, H. E. 1992. Mononuclear phagocytes as targets, tissue reservoirs, and immunoregulatory cells in human immunodeficiency virus disease. *Current Topics in Microbiology and Immunology* 181:239–263.

50. Meltzer, M. S., Nacy, C. A. 1989. Delayed type hypersensitivity and the induction of activated, cytotoxic macrophages. In: Paul, W. E., ed. 1989. *Fundamental Immunology*, Second Edition. New York: Raven Press, pp. 765–777.

51. Hans, S. L., Nottet, M,. de Graaf, L., de Vos, N. M., et al. 1993. Down-regulation of human immunodeficiency virus type 1 (HIV-1) production after stimulation of monocyte-derived macrophages infected with HIV-1. *Journal of Infectious Disease* 167:810–817.

52. Marshall, G. D., Gibbons, A. S., Purnell, L. S. 1993. Human cytokines induced by Acemannan. *Journal of Allergy and Clinical Immunology* 91:295 [abstract].

53. See: Tizard, I. R., Carpenter, R. H,. McAnalley, B. H., Kemp, M. C. 1989. The biological activities of mannans and related complex carbohydrates. *Molecular Biotherapy* 1:290–295; and Tizard, I. R. 1992. Immune stimulating carbohydrates. In: Roitt, I. M., ed. 1992. *Encyclopedia of Immunology.* San Diego, CA: Academic Press, Inc.

54. Cumberbatch, M., Gould, S. J., Peters, W., et al. 1992. Langerhans cells, antigen presentation and the diversity of responses to chemical allergens. *Journal of Investigative Dermatology* 99:107S–108S.

How DNCB Works

55. See: Gendelman, H. E., Morahan, P. S. 1992. Macrophages in viral infections. In: Lewis, C. E., O'D. Mcgee, J., eds. 1992. The *Macrophage.* New York: Oxford University Press, pp. 175–177.

56. The recent edition of *The Merck Manual* states the following: "Skin malignancies have regressed after induction of delayed hypersensitivity to dinitrochlorobenzene (DNCB) and subsequent direct application of DNCB to the tumor." Berkow, R., ed. 1992. *The Merck Manual of Diagnosis and Therapy.* Rathway, New Jersey: Merck Research Laboratories, p. 1292.

57. *The Illustrated Guide to Diagnostic Tests* states, "Skin tests employ new and recall antigens. New antigens—those not previously encountered by the patient, such as dinitrochlorobenzene (DNCB)—evaluate the patient's primary immune response when a sensitizing dose is given, followed by a challenge dose." Loeb, S., ed. 1993. *Illustrated Guide to Diagnostic Tests.* Springhouse, PA: Springhouse Corporation, pp. 1026–1030.

58. Meltzer, M. S., Nacy, C. A. 1989. Delayed type hypersensitivity and the induction of activated, cytotoxic macrophages. In: Paul, W. E., ed. 1989. *Fundamental Immunology,* Second Edition. New York: Raven Press, p. 775.

59. Meltzer, M. S., Nacy, C. A. 1989. Ibid, pp. 766–767.

DNCB Treatment Instructions

60. See: Gilden, D. 1993. DNCB Treatment Today. *AIDS Treatment News* 182:3–7.; and Hosein, S. 1993. Immunomodulators. *Treatment Update* 43:4(3):4–6.

Alternative Treatments for Herpes, Cytomegalovirus andVaricella Zoster Infections

61. Mann, J. A., Fowkes, S. W. 1983. *Wipe Out Herpes With BHT.* Manhattan Beach, CA: MegaHealth Society.

Chinese Herbs for HIV: A Critical Analysis

62. Li, X. Y. 1991. Immunomodulating Chinese herbal medicines. *Memorias Instituto Oswaldo Cruz* 86(S II):159–164.

63. See: Shearer, G., Clerici, M. 1992. T-helper immune dysfunction in HIV seropositive individuals: the role of Th1-Th2 cross regulation. *Chemical Immunology* 54:21–43; Janeway, C. A. 1993. How the Immune System Recognizes Invaders. *Scientific American* 269:72–79; and Paul, W. E. 1993. Infectious Diseases and the Immune System. Ibid. 269:90–97.

64. See: Sher, A., Coffman, R. L. 1992. Regulation of immunity to parasites by T-cells and T-cell-derived cytokines. *Annual Review of Immunology* 10:385–409; and Kaufmann, S. H. E. 1993. Immunity to intracellular bacteria. Ibid. 11:129–165.

65. Clerici, M., Shearer, G. 1993. A Th1→Th2 switch is a critical step in the etiology of HIV infection. *Immunology Today* 14:107–111.

66. Pamer, G. 1993. Cellular immunity to intracellular bacteria. *Current Opinion in Immunology* 5:492–496; Orme, I. M. 1993. Immunity to mycobacteria. Ibid. 5:497–502; Bancroft, G. J. 1993. the role of natural killer cells in innate resistance to infection. Ibid. 5:503–510; Modlin, R. L., Nutman, T. B. 1993. Type 2 cytokines and negative immune regulation in human infections. ibid. 5:511–517; James, S. L., Nacy,

C. 1993. Effector functions of activated macrophages against parasites. Ibid. 5:518–523; Reed, S. G., Scott, P. 1993. T-cell and cytokine responses in leishmaniasis. Ibid. 5:524–531; Subauste, C. S., Remington, J. S. 1993. Ibid. 5:532–537.

67. Roitt, I., Brostoff, J., Male, D., 1993. *Immunology,* Third Edition London: Mosby, p. 7.5

68. The recent edition of *The Merck Manual* states, "An increased incidence of lymphomas, particularly immunoblastic and undifferentiated or Burkitt types, has been seen in AIDS patients. Primary CNS involvement and disseminated disease have been reported. In about thirty percent of cases, the lymphomas are usually preceded by generalized lymphadenopathy, suggesting that polyclonal stimulation of B-cells results in the emergence of immortalized but not fully transformed B-cell clones. C-myc gene rearrangements are characteristic of AIDS-associated lymphomas. Response to modern therapy is posible, but toxicity is common and opportunistic infections continue to occur, resulting in short survival." Berkow, B., ed. 1992. *The Merck Manual of Diagnosis and Therapy.* Rathway: NJ: Merck Research Laboratories, p. 1248. See also: Levine, A. M. 1993. AIDS-related malignancies: the emerging epidemic. *Journal of the National Cancer Institute* 85:1382–1394.

69. See: Homsy, J., Meyer, Levy, J. A. 1990. Serum enhancement of human immunodeficiency virus (HIV) infection correlates with disease in HIV-infected individuals. *Journal of Virology* 64:1437–40; Dietrich, M. P., Ebenbichler, Marschang P., et al. 1993. HIV and human complement: mechanisms of interaction and biological implication. *Immunology Today* 14:435–440; and Spear, G. T. 1993. Interaction of non-antibody factors with HIV in plasma. *AIDS* 7:1149–1157

70. Zhao, K. S., Mancini, C., Doria, G. 1990. Enhancement of immune response in mice by Astragalus membranaceus extracts. *Immunopharmacology* 20:225–234.

71. Yeung, H. W., Cheung, K., Leung, K. N. 1982. Immunopharmacology of Chinese medicine 1, ginseng induced immunosuppression in virus-infected mice. *American Journal of Chinical Medicine* 10:44–54.

72. See: Pantaleo, G., Graziosi, C., Demarest, J. F., Butini, L., Montroni, M., Fox, C. H., Orenstein, J. M., Kotler, D. P., Fauci, A. S. 1993.

HIV infection is active and progressive in lymphoid tissue during the clinically latent stage of disease. *Nature* 362:355–358; and Fox, C. H., Cottler-Fox, M. 1992. The pathobiology of HIV infection. *Immunology Today* 13:353–356.

73. Tawfix, A. F., Bishop, S. J., Ayalp, A., el-Feraly, F. S. 1990. Effects of artemisinin dihydroartemisinin and arteether on immune response of normal mice. *International Journal of Immunopharmacology* 12:385–389.

74. See: Zhang, L. X., Yu, F. K., Zheng, Q. Y., et al. 1990. Immunosuppressive and antiinflammatory a. ctivities of tripterine. *Acta Pharmaceutica Sinica* 25:573–577; and Zheng, Y. L., Xu, Y., Lin, J. F. 1989. Immunosuppressive effects of wilfortrine and euonine. Ibid. 24:568–72.

75. Meltzer, M. S., Nacy, C. A. 1989. Delayed type hypersensitivity and the induction of activated, cytotoxic macrophages. In: Paul, W. E, ed. 1989. *Fundamental Immunology,* Second Edition. New York: Raven Press, pp. 765–777.

76. See: Roesler, J., Emmendorffer, A., Steinmuller, C., et al. 1991. Application of purified polysaccharides from cell cultures of the plant Echinacea purpurea to test subjects mediates activation of the phagocyte system. *International Journal of Immunopharmacology* 13:931–941; and Stimpel, M., Proksch, A., Wagner, H., Lohmann-Matthes, M. L. 1984. Macrophage activation and induction of macrophage cytotoxicity by purified polysaccharide fractions from the plant Echinacea purpurea. *Infection and Immunity* 46:845–849.

77. Hendler, S. S. 1990. *The Doctor's Vitamin and Mineral Encyclopedia.* New York, Fireside, pp. 293–294.

78. Xu-Amano, J., Kiyono, H., Jackson, R. J, et al. 1993. Helper T-cell subsets for Immunoglobulin A responses: oral immunization with tetanus toxoid and cholera toxin as adjuvant selectively induces Th2 cells in mucosa associated tissues. *Journal of Experimental Medicine* 178:1309–1320.

79. Liu, C. X., Xiao, P. G. 1992. Recent advances in ginseng research in China. *Journal of Ethnopharmacology* 36:27–38.

Glossary

Accessory cells: Lymphoid cells predominantly of the monocyte and macrophage lineage that cooperate with T- and B-lymphocytes in the formation of antibody and in other immune reactions.

Activated lymphocytes: Lymphocytes that have been stimulated by specific antigen or nonspecific mitogen.

Activated macrophages: Mature macrophages in a metabolic state caused by various stimuli, especially phagocytosis or lymphokine activity.

Acute phase proteins: Serum proteins whose levels increase during infection or inflammatory reactions.

Adaptive immunity: A series of host defenses characterized by extreme specificity and memory mediated by antibody or T-cells.

ADCC (antibody-dependent cell-mediated cytotoxicity): A form of lymphocyte-mediated cytotoxicity in which an effector cell kills an antibody-coated target cell, presumably by recognition of the Fc region of the cell-bound antibody through an Fc receptor present on the effector lymphocyte.

Adhesion: The 'sticking' of migratory leukocytes to endothelial or structural cells by the interaction of complementary adhesion proteins.

Adjuvant: A compound capable of potentiating an immune response.

Allergen: A foreign protein or hapten which induces the formation of anaphylactic antibodies and which may precipitate an allergic response.

Allergy (hypersensitivity): A disease or reaction caused by an immune response to one or more environmental antigens, resulting in tissue inflammation and organ dysfunction.

Allogeneic: Denotes the relationship that exists between genetically dissimilar members of the same species.

Anaphylaxis: A reaction of immediate hypersensitivity present in nearly all vertebrates that results from sensitization of tissue-fixed mast cells by cytotropic antibodies following exposure to antigen.

Anergy: A state of diminished or absent cell-mediated immunity as shown by the inability to react to a battery of common skin test antigens.

Antibody: A protein which is produced as a result of the introduction of an antigen and which has the ability to combine with the antigen that stimulated its production.

Antigen: A substance that reacts with antibodies or T-cell receptors evoked by immunogens.

Antigen processing: The conversion of an antigen by proteolysis into a form in which it can be recognized by lymphocytes.

Antigen-binding site: The part of an immunoglobulin that binds antigen.

Antigenic shift: Periodic changes over time in the surface antigens of certain viruses. These are caused by genetic mutations.

APCs (antigen-presenting cell): A cell that processes a protein antigen by fragmenting it into peptides that are presented on the cell surface in concert with class II major histocompatibility molecules for interaction with the appropriate T-cell receptor. B-cells, T-cells, dendritic cells, and macrophages can perform this function.

Atopy: A genetically determined state of hypersensitivity to common environmental allergens, mediated by IgE antibodies.

Attenuated: Rendered less virulent.

Autoantibody: Antibody to self antigens (autoantigens).

Autocrine: Effects of hormones on the cell that actually produces them.

Autoimmunity: Immunity to self antigens (autoantigens).

B-cells (also B-lymphocytes): B-cells are the bone-marrow derived precursors of plasma cells that produce antibody.

Basophils: A blood cell that has high-affinity receptors for IgE and generates inflammatory mediators in allergy.

BCG (bacillus Calmette-Guerin): A viable attenuated strain of Mycobacterium bovis that has been obtained by progressive reduction of virulence and that confers immunity to mycobacterial infection and possibly possesses anti-cancer activity in selected diseases.

Bystander lysis: Complement-mediated or cytokine-mediated lysis of cells in the immediate vicinity of an immune response, which are not themselves responsible for the activation. Also known as bystander effect.

Cachectin: A factor present in serum, which causes wasting and is identical to tumor necrosis factor alpha.

Carrier: An immunogenic substance that, when coupled to a hapten, renders the hapten immunogenic.

CD (cluster of differentiation): One or more cell surface molecules, detectable by monoclonal antibodies, that define a particular cell line or state of cellular differentiation.

Cell line: A collection of cells which divide continuously in culture. May be either monoclonal or polyclonal and may have been transformed naturally or be an artificial hybridization.

Cell cycle: The process of cell division which is divisible into four phases G1, S, G2 and M. DNA replicates during the S phase and the cell divides in the M (mitotic) phase.

Chemotaxis: Increased directional migration of cells particularly in response to concentration gradients of certain chemotactic factors.

Clonal abortion: Concept that the immune response of lymphocytes is curtailed by prevention of the further differentiation of immature cells.

Clonal anergy: Concept that the immune response is downregulated by lack of proliferation of effector and memory lymphocytes.

Clonal deletion: Concept that immune cells such as lymphocytes are physically deleted from the peripheral repertoire. Also known as programmed cell death or apoptosis.

Clonal selection: The fundamental basis of lymphocyte activation in which antigen selectively stimulates only those cells which express receptors for it to divide and differentiate.

Clone: A group of cells all of which are the progeny of a single cell.

CMI (cell-mediated immunity): A term used to refer to immune reactions that are mediated by cells, usually lymphocytes, rather than by antibody or other humoral factors.

Complement: A group of serum proteins involved in the control of inflammation, the activation of phagocytes and the lytic attack on cell membranes. The system can be activated by interaction with the immune system utilizing either the classical pathway (antibody-dependent) or alternate pathway (antibody-independent).

Conjugate: A combination of two molecules such as hapten and protein which can then become immunogenic and initiate an immune response.

Contact sensitivity: A type of delayed hypersensitivity reaction in which sensitivity to simple chemical compounds is manifested by skin reactivity.

Cytokines: A generic term for soluble molecules which mediate interactions between cells.

Cytophilic: Having a propensity to bind to cells.

Cytostatic: Having the ability to stop cell growth.

Cytotoxic: Having the ability to kill cells.

Dendritic cells: A set of antigen-presenting cells present in epithelial structures and in lymph nodes, spleen and at low levels in blood, which are particularly active in presenting antigen and stimulating T-cells.

Desensitization: A protocol of repeated injections of allergen or modified allergen with the aim of reducing a patient's allergic responsiveness to that antigen. Also known as hyposensitization.

Diapedesis: The movement of a blood leukocyte through a blood vessel wall into the extravascular compartment.

DTH (delayed-type hypersensitivity): This term includes the delayed skin reactions associated with Type IV hypersensitivity. A cell-mediated immune response producing a cellular infiltrate and edema that are maximal between 24 and 48 hours after antigen challenge.

Effector cells: A functional concept which in context means those lymphocytes or phagocytes which produce the end effect.

Endocrine: Effects of a hormone that are systemic.

Endocytosis: The process whereby material external to a cell is internalized within a particular cell. It consists of pinocytosis and phagocytosis.

Endothelium: Cells lining the blood vessels which contract to allow extravasation of plasma proteins and which express endothelial adhesion proteins.

Endotoxins: Lipopolysaccharides that are derived from the cell walls of gram-negative microorganisms and have toxic and pyrogenic effects when injected in vivo.

Enterotoxin: A heat-stable toxin produced by bacteria, which produces intestinal disease.

Eosinophils: Bone marrow derived granulocytes which are non-dividing granular cells with a limited life span in the circulation. They have both secretory and phagocytic functions and may play a specific role in defense against parasites.

Epitope: The simplest form of an antigenic determinant present on a complex antigenic molecule, which combines with antibody or T-cell receptor.

Exon: The coding segment of a DNA strand.

Exotoxins: Diffusible toxins produced by certain gram-positive and gram-negative microorganisms.

Fab: The part of an antibody molecule which contains the antigen-combining site, consisting of a light chain and part of the heavy chain; it is produced by enzymatic digestion.

Fc receptor: A receptor present on various subclasses of lymphocytes for the Fc fragment of immunoglobulins.

FDCs (follicular dendritic cells): Found in the secondary follicles of the B-cells areas of the lymph nodes and spleen. They present antigen to B-cells and lack class II MHC, but have complement receptors for interaction with immune complexes.

GALT (gut-associated lymphoid tissue): Refers to the accumulations of lymphoid tissue associated with the gastrointestinal tract.

Gamma globulins: Serum proteins with gamma mobility in electrophoresis that make up the majority of immunoglobulins and antibodies.

Generalized anaphylaxis: A shock-like state that occurs within minutes following an appropriate antigen-antibody reaction resulting from the systemic release of vasoactive amines.

Genome: The total genetic material from parents; not all of it is necessarily expressed in the individual.

Genotype: The genetic material inherited from parents; not all of it is necessarily expressed in the individual.

Germinal centers: A collection of metabolically active lymphoblasts, macrophages, and plasma cells that appears within the primary follicle of lymphoid tissues following antigenic stimulation.

Giant cells: Large multinucleated cells sometimes seen in granulomatous reactions and thought to result from the fusion of macrophages.

Granuloma: An organized structure of mononuclear cells that is the hallmark of cell-mediated immunity.

GVH (graft-versus-host) reaction: The clinical and pathologic seque-lae of the reactions of immunocompetent cells in a graft against the cells of the histoincompatible and immunodeficient recipient.

Haplotype: A set of genetic determinants located on a single chromosome.

Hapten: A small molecule which is incapable of inducing an anti-body response by itself but can, when bound to a protein carrier, act as an epitope, e.g., DNCB.

Helper (Th) cells: A functional subclass of T-cells which can help to generate cytotoxic T-cells and cooperate with B-cells in production of antibody response. Helper cells recognize antigen in association with class II MHC molecules.

Hematopoietic system: All tissues responsible for production of the cellular elements of peripheral blood. This term usually excludes strictly lymphocytopoietic tissue such as lymph nodes.

Histamine: A major vasoactive amine released from mast cell and basophil granules.

HLA (human leukocyte antigen): The major histocompatibility genetic region in humans. Class I MHC are HLA-A, B, C, and the class II MHC are HLA-DP, DQ, DR.

Homing receptors: Cell surface molecules that direct the cell to spe-cific locations in other organs or tissues.

Humoral: Pertaining to molecules in solution in a body fluid, partic-ularly antibody and complement.

Hyperreactivity: A state of increased reactivity to a provoking stimulus, e.g. bronchial hyperreactivity in asthma. Specifically, a greater mag-nitude of response to a given concentration of stimulus.

Hypersensitivity: Synonymous with allergy (by usage).

Hypogammaglobulinemia (agammaglobulinemia): A deficiency of all major classes of serum immunoglobulins.

Idiotope: An epitope (antigenic determinant) on an idiotype.

Idiotype: A unique antigenic determinant present on homogeneous antibody or myeloma protein. The idiotype appears to represent the antigenicity of the antigen-binding site of an antibody and is therefore located in the V region.

IFNs (interferons): A group of mediators which increase the resistance of cells to viral infection, and act as cytokines. IFN-γ is also an important immunological mediator that is particularly associated with cell-mediated immunity.

IL-1 to IL-13 (interleukins): Members of the cytokine family which were originally conceived as intercellular messengers between leukocytes but are now perceived as having wider immunological and inflammatory effects.

Immediate hypersensitivity: An antibody-mediated immunologic sensitivity that manifests itself by tissue reactions occurring within minutes after the antigen combines with its appropriate antibody.

Immune complexes: An aggregate of antibody and antigen which may induce a hypersensitivity response, often by stimulating the complement cascade.

Immune suppression: A variety of therapeutic maneuvers to depress or eliminate the immune response such as cyclosporine, FK-502, and corticosteroids.

Immune surveillance: A theory that holds that the immune system destroys tumor cells, which are constantly arising during the life of the individual.

Immunization: See Sensitization. Natural or artificial induction of an immune response, particularly when it renders the host protected from disease.

Immunogen: A substance that, when introduced into an animal, stimulates the immune response. The term immunogen may also denote a substance that is capable of stimulating an immune response, in contrast to a substance that can only combine with antibody, i.e., an antigen.

Immunoglobulin: All antibodies are immunoglobulins, but it is not certain that all immunoglobulins have antibody function.

Immunoglobulin class: A subdivision of immunoglobulin molecules based on unique antigenic determinants in the Fc region of the H chains. In humans there are 5 classes of immunoglobulins designated IgA, IgD, IgE, IgG, and IgM.

Immunoglobulin class switch: The process in which a B-cell precursor expressing IgM and IgG receptors differentiates into a B-cell producing IgA, IgE, or IgG antibodies without change in specificity for the antigenic determinant.

Immunoglobulin subclass: A subdivision of the classes of immunoglobulins based on structural and antigenic differences in the H chains. For human IgG there are 4 subclasses: IgG1, IgG2, IgG3, and IgG4.

Immunoglobulin supergene family: A structurally related group of genes that encode immunoglobulins, T-cell receptors, β2-microglobulin, and others.

Immunotherapy: Either hyposensitization in allergic diseases or treatment with immunostimulants or immunosuppressive drugs or biologic products. Also known as biological response modifiers (BRM).

Innate immunity: Various host defenses present from birth that do not depend on immunologic memory.

Inoculation: The introduction of an antigen or antiserum into an animal to confer immunity.

Introns: Noncoding regions of DNA interspersed among the exons.

K cell: A group of lymphocytes which are able to destroy their target by antibody-dependent cell-mediated cytotoxicity. They have Fc receptors.

Kinins: A group of vasoactive mediators produced following tissue injury.

Langerhans cells: Antigen-presenting cells of the skin which emigrate to local lymph nodes to become dendritic cells; they are very active in presenting antigen to T-cells.

Large granular lymphocytes (LGLs): a group of morphologically defined lymphocytes containing the majority of K cell and NK cell activity. They have both lymphocyte and monocyte/macrophage markers.

Lectin: A substance that is derived from a plant and has panagglutinating activity for erythrocytes. Lectins are commonly mitogens as well.

Leukotrienes: A collection of metabolites of arachidonic acid which have powerful pharmacological effects.

LFAs (leukocyte functional antigens): a group of three molecules which mediate intercellular adhesion between leucocytes and other cells in an antigen non-specific fashion.

Ligand: A linking (or binding) molecule.

Lipopolysaccharide (also endotoxin): A compound derived from a variety of gram-negative enteric bacteria that have various biologic functions including mitogenic activity for B-lymphocytes.

Locus: The specific site of a gene on a chromosome.

LPS (lipopolysaccharide): A product of some Gram-negative bacterial cell walls which can act as a polyclonal B-cell mitogen.

Lymphocyte: A mononuclear containing a nucleus with densely packed chromatin and a small rim of cytoplasm.

Lymphokines (also mediators of cellular immunity): A generic term for molecules other than antibodies which are involved in signaling between cells of the immune system and are produced by lymphocytes (e.g., interleukins, interferons, growth and stimulating factors).

Lymphotoxin (LT or TNF-β): A lymphokine that results in direct cytolysis following its release from stimulated lymphocytes.

Macrophages: Phagocytic mononuclear cells that derive from bone marrow monocytes and subserve accessory roles in cellular immunity.

MALT (mucosa-associated lymphoid tissue): Generic term of lymphoid tissue associated with the gastrointestinal tract, bronchial tree and other mucosa. This tissue produces a unique immunoglobulin (secretory IgA) and T-cell immunity for these mucosal surfaces.

Mast cell: A tissue cell that has high-affinity receptors for IgE and generates inflammatory mediators in allergy.

Membrane attack complex (MAC): The terminal complement components that, when activated, cause lysis of target cells.

MHC (major histocompatibility complex): A genetic region found in all mammals where products are primarily responsible for the rapid rejection of grafts between individuals, and function in signaling between lymphocytes and cells expressing antigen.

MHC class I: Histocompatibility antigen located on virtually all nucleated cells. Antigen is encoded in humans by A, B, and C loci. One of the encoded peptides is complexed with β2-microglobulin. The others are α1, α2, and α3.

MHC class II: Histocompatibility antigen expressed only on B-lymphocytes, macrophages, Langerhans/dendritic cells, endothelial cells, T-cells (on activation) and a few other cell types. Antigen is encoded in humans by DR, DP, and DQ loci. The encoded proteins are α1, α2, β1, and β2.

β2-Microglobulin: A protein that is associated with the outer membrane of many cells, including lymphocytes, and that functions as a structural part of the class I histocompatibility antigens on cells.

Mitogens: Substances which cause cells, particularly lymphocytes to undergo cell division.

MLR/MLC (mixed lymphocyte reaction/mixed lymphocyte culture): Assay system for T-cell recognition of allogeneic cells in which response is measured by proliferation in the presence of the stimulating cells.

Molecular mimicry: Immunologic cross-reactivity between determinants on an environmental antigen (such as a virus) and a self antigen, a notion that has been proposed to explain autoimmunity.

Monoclonal: Derived from a single clone, for example, monoclonal antibodies, which are produced by a single clone and are homogenous.

Mononuclear phagocyte system: Mononuclear cells found primarily in the reticular connective tissue of lymphoid and other organs that are prominent in chronic inflammatory states.

Mucosal homing: The ability of immunologically competent cells that arise from mucosal follicles to traffic back to mucosal areas.

Myeloma: A lymphoma produced from cells of the B-cell lineage.

Neoplasm: A synonym for cancerous tissue.

Neutralization: The process by which antibody or antibody in complement neutralizes the infectivity of microorganisms, particularly viruses.

Neutrophils: They perform many of the same phagocytic and degradative functions as macrophages.

NK (natural killer cells): A group of lymphocytes which have the intrinsic ability to recognize and destroy some virally infected cells and some tumor cells.

Nonresponder: A mammal unable to respond to an antigen, usually because of genetic factors.

Null cells: Cells lacking the specific identifying surface markers for either T-or B-lymphocytes.

Oncogene: A gene of either viral or mammalian origin that causes transformation of cells in culture.

Opportunistic infection: The ability of organisms of relatively low virulence to cause disease in the setting of altered immunity.

Opsonization: A process by which phagocytosis is facilitated by the deposition of opsonins (e.g., antibody and C3b) on the antigen.

Paracrine: Effects of a hormone that are only local.

Pathogen: An organism which causes disease.

Passive immunity: Protection achieved by introduction of preformed antibody or immune cells into a nonimmune host.

PCR (Polymerase chain reaction): A technique to amplify segments of genetic DNA or RNA of known composition with primers in sequential repeated steps.

Peripheral lymphoid organs: Lymphoid organs not essential to the ontogeny of immune responses, i.e., the spleen, lymph nodes, tonsils, and Peyer's patches.

Peyer's patches: Collections of lymphoid tissue in the submucosa of the small intestine that contain lymphocytes, plasma cells, germinal centers, and T-cell-dependent areas.

Phagocytes: Cells that are capable of ingesting particulate matter.

Phagocytosis: The process by which cells engulf material and enclose it within a vacuole (phagosome) in the cytoplasm.

Plasma cells: Fully differentiated antibody-synthesizing cells that are derived from B-lymphocytes.

Platelets (thrombocytes): In addition to their role in blood clotting, they are involved in the immune response especially in inflammation.

Primary lymphoid tissues: Lymphoid organs in which lymphocytes complete their initial maturation steps; they include the fetal liver, adult bone marrow and thymus, and bursa of Fabricius in birds.

Primary response: The immune response (cellular or humoral) following an initial encounter with a particular antigen.

Prime: To give an initial sensitization to antigen.

Prostaglandins: A variety of naturally occurring aliphatic acids with various biologic activities, including increased vascular permeability, smooth muscle contraction, bronchial constriction, and alteration in the pain threshold.

Pruritus: Localized skin itching caused by hypersensitivity reactions.

Pyrogens: Substances that are released either endogenously from leukocytes or administered exogenously, usually from bacteria, and that produce fever in susceptible hosts.

Radioimmunoassay: A variety of immunologic techniques in which a radioactive isotope is used to detect antigens or antibodies in some form of immunoassay.

Receptor: A cells surface molecule which binds specifically to particular extracellular molecules.

Respiratory burst: The process by which neutrophils and monocytes kill certain microbial pathogens by conversion of oxygen to toxic oxygen products.

Reticuloendothelial system: A diffuse system of phagocytic cells derived from the bone marrow stem cell which are associated with the connective tissue framework of the liver, spleen, lymph nodes and other serous cavities.

Retrovirus: A virus that contains and utilizes reverse transcriptase, e.g., human immunodeficiency virus or human T-cell leukemia virus.

Reverse transcriptase: An enzyme present in various microorganisms that catalyzes transcription of DNA from RNA rather than in the usual direction of transcription, which occurs from DNA to RNA.

Secondary response: The immune response which follows a second or subsequent encounter with a particular antigen.

Sensitization: The stimulation of allergic antibody production or delayed-type hypersensitivity by an initial encounter to a specific allergenic substance or hapten. Synonymous with primary response.

Serum sickness: An adverse immunologic response to a foreign antigen, usually a heterologous protein.

Slow virus: A virus that produces disease with a greatly delayed onset and protracted course such as HIV.

Somatic mutation: A process occurring during B-cell maturation and affecting the antibody gene regions, which permits refinement of antibody specificity.

Suppressor T-cells: A subset of T-lymphocytes that suppress antibody synthesis by B-cells or inhibit other cellular immune reactions by effector T-cells. This suppressor function is presently believed to be controlled by cytokines.

Synergism: Cooperative interaction.

T-cell (T-lymphocyte): A thymus-derived cell that participates in a variety of cell-mediated immune reactions; common usage is T4 or CD4 and T8 or CD8.

TCR (T-cell receptor): The T-cell antigen receptor consisting of either an αβ dimer (TCR-2) or a γδ dimer (TCR-1) associated with the CD3 molecular complex.

T-dependent/T-independent: T- dependent antigens require immune recognition by both T- and B-cells to produce an immune response. T-independent antigens can directly stimulate B-cells to produce specific antibody.

Th1-cells: A subdivision of helper T-cells involved in cell-mediated immunity and characterized by their production of IFN-γ, and IL-2. The cytotoxic T-cells involved in this response are known as T1.

Th2-cells: A subdivision of T-helper-cells involved in allergy and other antibody responses by their influence of B-cells to produce IgE, IgG and proinflammatory effects. Characterized by their production of IL-4, IL-5, IL-6 and IL-10. The suppressor T-cells involved in this response are known as T2.

Thymus: The central lymphoid organ that is present in the thorax and controls the ontogeny of T-lymphocytes.

Thymus-dependent antigen: Antigen that depends on T-cell interaction with B-cells for antibody synthesis, e.g., erythrocytes, serum proteins, and hapten-carrier complexes.

Thymus-independent antigen: Antigen that can induce an immune response without the apparent participation of T-lymphocytes.

TNF (tumor necrosis factor): A cytokine released by activated macrophages that is structurally related to lymphotoxin released by activated T-cells.

Tolerance: Traditionally denotes that condition in which responsive cell clones have been eliminated or inactivated by prior contact with antigen, with the result that no immune response occurs on administration of antigen.

Transcription: The synthesis of RNA molecules from a DNA template.

Translation: The process of formation of a peptide chain from individual amino acids to form a protein molecule.

Tumor-specific antigens: Cell surface antigens that are expressed on malignant but not normal cells.

Urticaria (hives): Localized edematous pruritic skin plaques caused by hypersensitivity reactions.

Vaccination: Immunization with antigens administered for the prevention of infectious diseases (term originally coined to denote immunization against vaccinia or cowpox virus).

Weal: An area of edema produced at the site of intradermal introduction of allergen, histamine or similar provocant. Stimulation of axon reflexes in the weal area gives rise to the larger flare response.

Xenogeneic: Denotes the relationship that exists between members of genetically different species.

Resource Guide

ACEMANNAN *see also DeVeras Beverage*

For more information on Acemannan, contact Carrington Laboratories, 2001 Walnut Hill Lane, Irving, Texas, 75038; (214) 518-1300.

BOOKS & WRITTEN MATERIALS

Tom O'Connor's book *Living With Aids* and many other written resources can be reviewed at the Healing Alternatives Foundation, 1748 Market Street, San Francisco, CA 94102; (415) 626-4053 or 626-2316.

CHINESE MEDICINE

For more information on Chinese Medicine or treatment options, contact Quan Yin Clinic, 1748 Market Street, San Francisco, CA 94102; (415) 861-4964.

COMPUTER INFORMATION NETWORKS

For more information on HIV/AIDS Info BBS, or other AEGIS Network Affiliates, contact the Sisters of St. Elizabeth of Hungary, Attn: AIDS/HIV Info BBS, P.O. Box 184, San Juan Capistrano, CA 92693-0184; or call the BBS number: (714) 248-2836

DEVERAS BEVERAGE *see also Acemannan*

The DeVeras Beverage may be purchased by sending a check/money order for $160.00 for a case of sixteen bottles (an eight-week supply) to DeVeras, Inc., 3404 Greenville Avenue, Suite 104, Dallas, TX, 75206; (800) 659-4619; (214) 823-4659. The company makes no medical claims for this product, and can only provide information on ordering.

DNCB

Information on DNCB can be obtained from the DNCB Hotline: (415) 954-8896.

DNCB can be obtained from DNCB Treatment Issues, 2261 Market Street, #499, San Francisco, CA 94114. An initial supply of four bottles with an information packet costs $20.00 (including shipping). Individual bottles are $5.00 each and should last six months.

DNCB is also available from the Healing Alternatives Foundation, 1748 Market Street, San Francisco, CA 94102; (415) 626-4053 or 626-2316. An initial supply of four bottles with treatment instructions costs $20.11, plus $5.00 shipping. Individual bottles are $4.31 each, plus $5.00 shipping, and should last six months.

HYPERICIN

Ten-milligram capsules of pure hypericin can be obtained from Pacific Biologicals (800)869-8783 at a cost of $65.00 for fifteen ten-milligram capsules. This company's pricing structure is currently under review, so the cost may be reduced shortly.

A product of similar quality at a competitive price may be purchased from the LIFELINK Buyer's Club, (805) 473-1389.

MEMBRANE FLUIDIZERS

A high neutral lipid egg lecithin product made by Jarrow is available at a cost of approximately $90.00 for 100 ten-gram doses. Contact the Healing Alternatives Foundation-Buyers Club, 1748 Market Street, San Francisco, CA 94102; (415) 626-5053 or 626-2316.

A comparable, and more economical, version of the membrane fluidizing treatment can be produced at home using a soy lecithin extract called PC-55 manufactured by Twinlabs. Twenty ten-gram doses can be made by combining ten tablespoons of the PC-55 granules and twenty-four tablespoons of water in a bowl. Slowly add exactly twelve and one-half tablespoons of butter (measured before melting) and whip the mixture thoroughly for five minutes. Divide into twenty even doses; two ice cube trays can be used for this purpose and for storage. To improve taste, whip the substance in a blender with fruit juice. This treatment must be taken on an empty stomach, and fats should be avoided for two hours after consumption. For CMV treatment, at least two doses daily are recommended.

TREATMENT INFORMATION

For the most objective and reliable information on promising AIDS-related treatments, we highly recommend *Treatment Update,* a publication of CATIE (Community AIDS Treatment Information Exchange). Yearly subscription rates are $15.00 for individuals and $25.00 for institutions. To subscribe, send a check or money order (payable in U.S. dollars only) to CATIE, 517 College Street, Suite 324, Toronto, Ontario, Canada M6G 4A2; (800) 263-1638. No one will be denied a subscription due to lack of funds.